THE FIRST YEAR™

Scleroderma

An Essential Guide for the Newly Diagnosed

KAREN GOTTESMAN was diagnosed with scleroderma in 1999. She currently serves on the local board of directors in Los Angeles, and is the former education chairperson in charge of both physician and patient education, for the Southern California chapter of the Scleroderma Foundation. She lives with her family in Pacific Palisades, California.

THE COMPLETE FIRST YEAR™ SERIES

The First Year—Type 2 Diabetes by Gretchen Becker
The First Year—IBS by Heather Van Vorous
The First Year—Hepatitis C by Cara Bruce and Lisa Montanarelli
The First Year—Fibroids by Johanna Skilling
The First Year—Hepatitis B by William Finley Green
The First Year—Crohn's Disease and Ulcerative Colitis by Jill Sklar
The First Year—Multiple Sclerosis by Margaret Blackstone
The First Year—Hypothyroidism by Maureen Pratt
The First Year—HIV by Brett Grodeck
The First Year—Fibromyalgia by Claudia Craig Marek
The First Year—Lupus by Nancy C. Hanger
The First Year—Scleroderma by Karen Gottesman

THE FIRST YEAR™

Scleroderma

An Essential Guide for the Newly Diagnosed

Karen Gottesman

Foreword by Daniel E. Furst, M.D.

MARLOWE & COMPANY ■ NEW YORK

Published by
Marlowe & Company
An Imprint of Avalon Publishing Group Incorporated
245 West 17th Street • 11th Floor
New York, NY 10011-5300

Library of Congress Cataloging-in-Publication Data
Gottesman, Karen, 1961–
    The first year—scleroderma : an essential guide for the
newly diagnosed / Karen Gottesman ; foreword by Daniel
E. Furst.
        p. cm. — (The first year series)
Includes index.
    ISBN 1-56924-439-1
    1. Scleroderma (Disease) 2. Patient education. I. Title:
Scleroderma. II. Title. III. Series.

RL451.G68 2004
    616.5'44—dc22   2003061517

9 8 7 6 5 4 3 2 1

Designed by Pauline Neuwirth,
    Neuwirth and Associates, Inc.

Printed in the United States of America

Distributed by Publishers Group West

For Maya and Evan,
my true source of inspiration.

"In three words,
I can sum up everything
I learned about life:
It goes on."
—Robert Frost

Contents

Foreword

by Daniel E. Furst, M.D.

SCLERODERMA CAN BE a devastating disease, particularly when you first hear the word, as many people perceive it as unknown, un-understood, and untreatable. It is, in fact, true that there remains a lot to learn about this disease. Fortunately, in the last 15 to 20 years, a great deal has been learned about its pathogenesis and natural history as well as its measurement. Most encouraging, more and more treatments are actively being developed.

This book explains a good deal of the above background. It is laid out in terms of your day-to-day, week-to-week, and month-to-month questions. It could be read from cover to cover, but its layout encourages you to read several chapters at a time and does not force you to treat this as the usual dry textbook. As well as discussing scleroderma and its manifestations, it takes you through the many questions you may have regarding scleroderma. In important and unusual ways, it asks the "real" questions that patients have, including less-often-discussed issues such as physical changes; depression and how to deal with it; significant work issues; and issues relating to disability, alternative therapies, sex, and pregnancy.

There are other books on scleroderma that are good in their own ways, but this book is probably the most patient-oriented book that has yet been published.

An important part of this book is its easy and readable style and its very thorough index, which allows you to look up those areas that concern you TODAY. And it gives general facts and approaches that are logical and thorough without overburdening you with every twist and turn and every tiny detail of each of the many facets of this disease. This book will help you, your family, your friends, and your other supporters deal with a difficult and chronic illness, while at the same time encouraging you to take control of your life.

DANIEL E. FURST, M.D.
Carl M. Pearson Professor of Rheumatology
David Geffen School of Medicine at the University of California
Los Angeles, California

Introduction

SCLERODERMA IS perhaps one of the most complicated and perplexing conditions for both doctors and patients
alike. Although it can affect just about every system in the body,
no two patients are affected in the same way. To add to the
complexity of the disease, scleroderma comes in many different forms. Some types are merely an inconvenience; other types
can be life-threatening. And it can be incredibly difficult to
diagnose. Although scleroderma has been around since the late
1800s, criteria for the classification of systemic sclerosis (scleroderma) by the American College of Rheumatology didn't
come about until 1980. Perhaps the most famous person to
develop scleroderma was the artist Paul Klee. As a pioneer of
modern art, Klee's whimsical and vivid paintings became world-
famous. But even Klee was misdiagnosed at first. He was initially diagnosed with the measles, only to find out later he was
really suffering from systemic scleroderma. As his disease worsened, it was reflected in both the tone and color of his paintings. Although bitterness, fear, and grief dominated his
paintings in the year before his death, it was also the year his
productivity increased. He painted over 1,200 paintings that

year; more than ever before in one year. He was known for his positive view of life, and perhaps his surge of productivity represented hope. Because even with a diagnosis of scleroderma, one must never lose hope. Since Klee's death in 1940, much has changed. Although we still have a long way to go, the advancement of science has allowed us to come up with better treatments and better ways to diagnose scleroderma. I know. I have scleroderma and realize how far we've come and how much more we need to learn about it.

What happened to me

The early signs of scleroderma can often be so vague, you may not even think there's anything wrong. Or seriously wrong, anyway. That's how my disease started. My first symptom involved my esophagus. I began to notice a problem swallowing my food. My food seemed to be getting stuck in my esophagus, and I needed large quantities of water to push it down. At first, the problem was fairly transient. And it seemed to be happening mostly with foods tougher to swallow, like meats and breads. But then it got progressively worse, and I began having problems with softer foods as well. Not one to worry too much about my health, I continued on like that for several months, while subconsciously eliminating the foods I couldn't swallow from my diet. On a routine visit to my physician, I casually mentioned my swallowing problem and he recommended I see a gastroenterologist right away. The gastroenterologist ran a few tests and was baffled as to the cause. He gave me a few different medications to try and when they all failed, he told me there wasn't anything else he could do for me. He more or less dismissed me as a patient. Although I was a bit perturbed at his dismissal of me, it wasn't until much later in the process that I realized how typical his behavior was in the search for a diagnosis.

My next symptom didn't occur until many months later, after a bad bout with the flu. This particular flu had left me with such a horrendous cough that it sent me right back to my internist . . . again. After a routine X ray, I was diagnosed with bronchitis and given a prescription for some antibiotics. Being the compliant patient that I am, I finished the course of antibiotics and waited patiently to get better. And waited, and waited, and waited. By the time I went back to my doctor a month later, not only was my cough worse, but I had been hit with the most overwhelming fatigue I had ever felt. My doctor chalked it up to the life of a working mom with two toddlers at home and gave me another course of antibiotics. He said if I wasn't better in a few weeks, to come back in for a recheck. I continued working as my cough worsened. Those I worked with just shook their heads when they heard me cough and were concerned I might have pneumonia or perhaps even tuberculosis. Because I had just had a bout with pneumonia the year before, I thought it prudent to go back to my doctor to get checked out again. Only this time, I had a brand-new symptom: My fingers were going numb.

At this point, I found it incredibly coincidental that I would be experiencing such strange symptoms all at the same time. First it was my esophagus, then my lungs, and now my fingers. After giving it some thought, I became certain that all these symptoms were somehow related. More concerned than usual, I presented my new symptom to my doctor and told him my thoughts about how these symptoms must somehow all be connected. I was sure he would be able to connect the dots for me. Boy, was I wrong. Not only did he discount my theory, he told me it was impossible for my symptoms to be related because each problem was an isolated incident caused by something different. But he had no idea what any of the causes were. And that was that. No further tests, no nothing. Then he promptly sent me to a neurologist about my numb fingers. At this point, other symptoms began popping up as well. My joints became horribly achy, and I developed enormous bruises on my body. My GI symptoms now included my intestines and I could hardly eat. I continued to lose weight and began to feel faint all the time. I felt like I was falling apart. Then I went to see the neurologist. And that visit turned out to be the turning point for me. After he ruled out MS or any other type of neurological problem as the cause of my symptoms, he indeed *was* convinced that all my symptoms were related. He recommended I see a rheumatologist.

Here's where my story may begin to sound quite familiar. As my health continued to decline, I was shuffled from specialist to specialist, each uncovering another problem yet unable to give me a proper diagnosis. The rheumatologist had taken lots of blood on my first appointment but had gotten inconclusive results. Although my labs indicated many abnormalities (which is a strange blessing in disguise, as many patients who go through this same process have completely normal labs and are often told their symptoms are all in their head or are caused by stress), the rheumatologist was hesitant to give me a diagnosis without waiting a bit longer to see how things evolved. He thought, due to some of my lab results, that I might have lupus, but he nevertheless wanted to play the waiting game. And that meant being patient and doing absolutely nothing until I had an official diagnosis. After eight long months, no treatment, no nothing.

Well, I wasn't quite so patient. At this point, my oxygen levels were falling and I was now going back and forth between a cardiologist and a pulmonologist trying to figure out whether the problem was with my lungs or my heart. And each specialist blamed the other organ. By now, my GI tract had completely stopped working from my esophagus down to my lower intestine. Plus, the pain from my joints was getting worse and the fatigue was unrelenting. Not only did I want some answers, I wanted some relief. I decided to see a new rheumatologist, who concluded it was indeed some type of an overlap syndrome (lupus and scleroderma) and said he would begin treatment immediately. Finally! He explained that, when a patient exhibits symptoms from more than one type of connective-tissue disease, the condition can either stay permanently mixed, or it can evolve into one particular disease (like lupus *or* scleroderma). But regardless of which disease I had, he was going to treat the symptoms. What a relief! I was thrilled to have finally found such a competent doctor. Unfortunately, my excitement was short-lived. Because my case became so complicated with multi-organ involvement, my lovely, new, competent doctor recommended I see a new rheumatologist who had more experience in treating complex cases. Although I was frustrated initally at having to change doctors again, I realized this was the best piece of advice I had received since my ordeal began. Not only did I respect my doctor for admitting he was in over his head, but I found he had sent me to an excellent diagnostician, who eventually was able to give me my official diagnosis.

As my disease rolled out over the next year or so, it became apparent, through many months of testing on just about every organ in my body, that I had scleroderma. And although I also tested positive to antibodies found in lupus, my disease was predominantly scleroderma, sans the hallmark of the disease: skin involvement. Had I had any skin involvement, my diagnosis probably could have been made a lot sooner. The good news was that at least I knew what I had, but the bad news was that my condition continued to deteriorate. In an effort to stabilize my disease, I tried treatment after treatment—to no avail. And then I began to do some serious research.

I was determined to fight this thing and win, but I needed more knowledge to help me with my battle. And so the story begins.

How to use this book

Getting a diagnosis of scleroderma is not only overwhelming, it can be downright shocking. But once the shock has faded, what most patients seem to have in common is their need for more information. You may have picked up this book right around the time of your diagnosis, or perhaps you're still going through the diagnostic process. Wherever you are in your journey, the same advice applies: Use this book at your own pace. Whether you have localized scleroderma or systemic scleroderma, you'll find a broad range of information that basically has some use for everyone.

The format of this book is set up to take you through your first year of diagnosis, first day by day, then week by week, and finally month by month. The first few days will help you learn the ABCs of your new disease. In the beginning, it may be best to start out slowly so you don't overwhelm yourself. Each day, week, and month is divided into a Living section and a Learning section. The Living section deals with the factual issues relating to scleroderma. It includes information on topics such as medical tests, clinical trials, job-related issues, and alternative therapies. The Learning section focuses on disease-related issues. Some people may want to read the information all at once; others may like to browse. Feel free to go at your own pace and skip to those chapters that are of the most interest to you right now. Also, the terms in **boldface** are defined in the glossary at the end of this book.

I will not prescribe

I am not a doctor. I will not prescribe for you. While I will provide you with a broad overview of treatments available right now, I will by no means tell you which is the best treatment for you. That's between you and your doctor. There are as many different types of scleroderma as there are treatment philosophies and strategies. What works for one person with one type of scleroderma may not work for another. And most likely won't. This is a complicated disease with the possibility of multi-organ system involvement.

No two people are affected in the same way. And that means no two people are treated the same way, either. Use the information provided in this book as a guide to make you aware of what options are available to you right now. As research continues to evolve, keep in mind that treatments will change as well. It's up to you to remain an informed and educated patient so that you can make the best decisions for your long-term health.

Where the focus is

The focus of this book is to help you become an active, educated participant in your own health care. To do that, you need to learn all you can about your new disease. Learning the language of scleroderma is crucial to making informed decisions about your care, but knowing you are not alone can make all the difference in how you feel on a daily basis. The diagnosis of a rare, chronic disease can leave you feeling very vulnerable. This book allows you to explore ways to feel more confident in your new role as a patient, while educating you about scleroderma along the way. You can use as much or as little of the information as you need. You're the one in control. You decide what you need to know and when you need to know it. You'll learn some hard facts about scleroderma in Days 1 and 2, so keep in mind it may be overwhelming to digest it all at once. Take it slowly and go at your own pace. Remember, you can always come back to it.

Some of the chapters (such as Month 3, which talks about clinical trials, or Month 9, which talks about pregnancy) may only apply to certain people; other chapters will provide information that's applicable to all patients. Throughout the book, you'll also find comments and experiences from real scleroderma patients. As a patient, I often found it helpful to read about other scleroderma patients' experiences. I hope you do, too.

Keep on learning

This book is only the beginning of a lifelong learning process. By the end of your first year with scleroderma, you should have a substantial education, which you will hopefully continue building on for years to come. And share with others. One of the best ways to keep on learning is to get involved in your local scleroderma community. Not only will getting involved allow you to meet others and share experiences, it will also help keep you informed of current treatment developments and efforts toward a cure. Scleroderma can be a very tricky disease. You must try your best to stay one step ahead of it. Whether through the Internet, your doctor, medical journals, or other sources, do whatever you can to remain an informed and educated patient. And hopefully, this book will become a long-term resource tool for you to use again and again. If anything, it will continue to remind you that you are not alone on this journey—you're in good company.

Devastating Bombshell or Tremendous Relief?

WHETHER YOU were expecting a diagnosis of scleroderma or not, actually receiving one is enough to send even the most prepared patient into a state of shock. This is completely normal. No one likes to hear that he or she has a rare, chronic, incurable disease, especially one he or she has probably never before heard of. Your journey to your diagnosis may have taken years. Or maybe it came out of the blue. But no matter how it came about, the feelings are the same: shock, fear, panic, and disbelief. And then the questions start: Why me? What have I done wrong?

Getting scleroderma is not your fault

Let's get a few things straight. First of all, stop questioning yourself. You didn't do anything wrong. Getting scleroderma is not your fault. You didn't "do" anything to cause your disease. But you're not alone in thinking this way. For now, you need to concentrate on adjusting to the news of your diagnosis. Your goal is to learn to accept your diagnosis, but keep in mind that usually doesn't happen overnight. For most, it's a gradual process that begins on the first day of diagnosis. Sometimes, it takes years for the news to sink in. Valerie was diagnosed two years ago. Even after going through a yearlong diagnostic process as well as dealing with the disease for more than two years, Valerie says the news has yet to sink in. Although the initial panic has subsided, she still has a hard time accepting the fact that she has a chronic disease. It's okay to take as much time as you need in accepting your diagnosis—just as long as you don't neglect your health during your quest to come to terms with the truth.

Finally, a diagnosis

The reality is, most of you have probably been waiting for this day for a long time. You've been feeling ill for quite some time and have been shuffling back and forth from doctor to doctor in search of answers. Due to its complexity, scleroderma can be incredibly difficult to diagnose. Not only does diagnosis involve differentiating it from other connective-tissue diseases, it also involves identifying the particular type that you have. And that can take years. Shirley's diagnosis took four years and four doctors. She was incredibly relieved to have a diagnosis—"but not that one," she says wistfully. Bonnie D's diagnosis took two years and two doctors. She was also relieved to finally get a diagnosis, because she was tired of her doctors treating her like a hypochondriac. Lydia's diagnosis took nine months and three doctors. She had done some research on her own ahead of time and suspected the cause, but she was nonetheless relieved to finally have a name for her symptoms. Linda, on the other hand, was completely "blindsided" by her diagnosis. While she had been experiencing some very vague symptoms like fatigue and malaise, she was diagnosed on a routine appointment for something completely unrelated. She was shocked. Christie was also shocked by her diagnosis. She hadn't experienced a single symptom except for **Raynaud's phenomenom**.

According to scleroderma specialists, the average scleroderma patient sees anywhere from two to five doctors before receiving the diagnosis. (And, as you can see from the stories above, it can take just as many years.) The reality of actually hearing your diagnosis comes either as a complete shock or an enormous relief. Either way, the end result is the same: You've been diagnosed with a disease you're going to have for the rest of your life. And those are hard words to hear.

Scleroderma is a different disease for everyone

Scleroderma comes in many different types and can vary greatly in severity. For some, it's merely a nuisance; for others it can be life-threatening. To add to its complexity, no two patients are affected in the same way. Some people hear the word *incurable* and begin to panic. Don't. Just because there is no cure for scleroderma doesn't mean there aren't treatments. One of the most frustrating things you'll find about scleroderma is its unpredictability. That alone can wreak havoc on your emotional stability. Some diseases run a fairly predictable course, but scleroderma's not one of them. My own experience with the disease has been anything but predictable. Especially during the first year. But even with all its unpredictability, you *can* learn to live well with scleroderma. It all begins with educating yourself about your disease and learning to become your own advocate. It's easy right now to feel very intimidated by scleroderma. You're entering a world you've never experienced before. The terminology, the doctor appointments, the medical tests, not to mention the emotional rollercoaster you're on—no wonder you feel so overwhelmed. But learning about your new disease will allow you to feel more in control. It also allows you to make informed decisions about your health care. And although it necessitates learning a whole new language, I think you'll be happy you did, in the long run.

Beginning your journey

Being diagnosed with a disease that has no cause or cure is a life-changing experience. And your life as you know it is about to change. The good news is that your journey toward a diagnosis is finally over. Now, a new journey is about to begin. Preparing for a journey can be stressful. And this type of journey is no different. But, the better prepared you are for any journey, the more smoothly it seems to go. You have a lot to learn about your new disease. Let's get started.

IN A SENTENCE:

> *Whether you're relieved or shocked by your diagnosis, the most important thing to remember is, getting scleroderma is not your fault.*

learning

It's Spelled
S-C-L-E-R-O-D-E-R-M-A

SO, YOU'VE just been diagnosed with a rare, chronic disease you've never heard of, let alone can spell or pronounce. The name alone is pretty scary. For many years, my young son thought I had a disease called *sclerogerma*. The name somehow seemed so descriptive and appropriate for the disease at the time, I never bothered to correct him. Not for several years anyway. Although it may be hard to get used to this strange-sounding disease in the beginning, you will become much more comfortable with the name as you start to learn exactly what the disease is all about. And at the very least, you'll learn how to spell its name.

The name *scleroderma* comes from the Greek word *sklerosis*, which means hardness, and *derma* which means skin. In essence, scleroderma literally means hard skin. Though usually referred to as a single disease, scleroderma comes in many forms and is divided into several different types. You'll learn more about these types in Day 2. I remember when I was first diagnosed with scleroderma, the few people who had heard of it would say, "Oh, scleroderma, that's like skin cancer, right?" Or, "Isn't that a lot like eczema?" Their responses made me realize how many misconceptions there are about the disease. Unfortunately, many of those misconceptions are held by members of the medical profession, as well. I can't count the number of times I've had to correct one specialist or another on misinformation they've had about scleroderma. You'll find the more you know about your disease, the more control you'll have over your own treatment and care. You'll learn more about how to begin educating yourself in Day 6.

Scleroderma is classified in many different ways

When you are first diagnosed, one of your questions will probably be, What type of disease is scleroderma? The answer tends to be a bit complicated, so let's break it down step by step.

1. ***Scleroderma is an autoimmune disease.*** Although some research indicates that scleroderma may not fit the traditional model of an **autoimmune disease**, it is still categorized as one. An autoimmune disease is a disease in which the immune system attacks the body's own tissue. For some reason, the immune system becomes misdirected and begins to attack the very organs it was designed to protect. In scleroderma, the activation of the immune system causes damage to two main areas: the small blood vessels and the collagen-producing cells located throughout the entire body. The problem in scleroderma is that the cells start producing **collagen** as if there were an injury somewhere in the body, even though no injury has occurred. Collagen is a fibrous protein in the body that provides firmness in the skin and forms the lining of the organs. It is the basic structural protein in the bones, tendons, ligaments, and joints. In milder forms of the disease, the effects of this collagen buildup are limited to the skin and the blood vessels. In more serious forms, the excess collagen interferes with the normal functioning of the skin, blood vessels, joints, and internal organs such as the lungs, kidneys, and GI tract.

2. ***Scleroderma is a rheumatic disease.*** A rheumatic disease refers to a group of conditions characterized by **inflammation**, with or without pain, in the muscles, joints, or fibrous tissue.

3. ***Scleroderma is a connective-tissue disease.*** Often referred to as a collagen vascular disease, a connective-tissue disease affects the major substances in the skin, tendons, and bones.

No, you don't have three separate diseases. But you do have a disease that falls under many different categories. Now you're beginning to understand why there's so much confusion surrounding the disease. When Bev was first diagnosed, she picked up an old medical manual that said, "Scleroderma is a grave disease that turns your body to stone." She was horrified. Be careful what you read. And make sure the information is current. Getting a diagnosis of scleroderma is scary enough without having to contend with all the wild descriptions and misconceptions out there.

Criteria for the classification of scleroderma

In 1980, the American College of Rheumatology came up with criteria that must be present in order to receive an official diagnosis of systemic scleroderma. A patient must have one major criterion or at least two minor criteria to be diagnosed with the systemic form of the disease. The localized form is excluded from these criteria.

MAJOR CRITERION
- Typical sclerodermatous skin changes: tightness, thickening, and non-pitting induration on the fingers and hands (skin thickening may also affect other parts of the extemities *in addition* to the fingers and hands)

MINOR CRITERIA
- Sclerodactyly (skin thickness of the fingers)
- Digital pitting scars
- Bibasilar pulmonary **fibrosis**

Although it's easy to get caught up in the "Do I fit the criteria?" mode, try not to. Other variables often come into play, as well. Let your doctor be the one to assess your situation and figure out whether you meet the criteria or not.

Who gets scleroderma?

GENDER

Although scleroderma does occur in men and children, most scleroderma patients are women. In fact, female patients outnumber malepatients 4 to 1. According to the National Institutes of Health (NIH), by the middle to late childbearing years (30–55), women develop scleroderma at a rate 7 to 12 times higher than men. And 80 percent of those diagnosed with systemic scleroderma (the more serious form) are women.

CHILDREN

Localized scleroderma, the milder form of the disease, is more common in children. Some children do develop systemic disease, but this happens much less frequently. When scleroderma does occur in children, it is called juvenile scleroderma and is treated by a pediatric **rheumatologist**.

ETHNICITY

African Americans tend to have a slightly higher risk of getting the disease, especially when they're younger. They tend to develop the systemic form of scleroderma more often than Caucasians; the reason for this is unclear.

GEOGRAPHY

According to the Scleroderma Foundation, there are an estimated 300,000 people in the United States. who have scleroderma. This number appears to be higher than in Europe or Japan; however, this may be due in part to the differences in the methods of counting cases. Another reason for the difference is that scleroderma is so often misdiagnosed or undiagnosed, thus causing confusion in estimating the number of those afflicted with the disease.

What causes scleroderma?

Although much research is focused on the answer to this question, the cause of scleroderma is unknown. It is thought that some people may have a genetic predisposition to scleroderma. However, this gene or combination of genes does not actually cause scleroderma. It merely puts you at greater risk of getting scleroderma. Other factors need to be present to initiate the disease process.

The scleroderma gene

According to the NIH, genes seem to put certain people at risk for the disease, but scleroderma is not passed from parent to child, as with some **genetic** diseases. Some diseases, like scleroderma, can occur from an interaction between an external trigger and an internal genetic predisposition. Suspected environmental triggers include viral infections, certain adhesive and coating materials, and some organic solvents. Now, before you go playing junior detective in search of a cause for your disease, remember this: Scientists have been working on this question for decades. Be patient. One day, we will have an answer.

IN A SENTENCE:

Scleroderma, typically classified as an autoimmune disease, affects mostly women and has no known cause or cure.

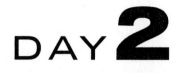

living

What You Need to Know Right Now

YOU'RE STILL reeling from your diagnosis. Your mind is racing and you're not sure what to do next. There's so much you want to know about scleroderma but you're wondering where to start. It all seems overwhelming. This is a normal reaction. But, before you inundate yourself with the hard facts of your new disease, let's start with some of the basic issues you need to know right now. You'll have plenty of time to learn the hard facts later.

Just the basics

You are not contagious. This is not like the flu. You can't catch it or give it to others. You can still kiss your spouse, hug your kids, and pet your dog. Although scientists don't know the exact cause of scleroderma, they do know it's not transmittable. When those around you find out you were just diagnosed with a new disease, they may be concerned for their own health. Especially if it's a disease they've never heard of. Tell them to relax. As much as you'd like to give your disease away, you can't.

But you *can* begin to educate others on scleroderma. It's an excellent way to create awareness for your new disease.

You don't have cancer. You don't even have a distant relative of cancer. Cancer, as defined by the American Cancer Society, is a group of diseases defined by uncontrolled growth and spread of abnormal cells. You do not have a tumor. There is no malignancy growing inside of you. You have a connective-tissue disease. And cancer is, well, cancer.

You are not alone. Although you may feel alone, you're not. You are among 300,000 other people who have felt the exact same way you're feeling right now. Shock, fear, isolation—these are all normal feelings to be having. You'll learn more about how to cope with these feelings in Day 7. For now, take some comfort in knowing you are not alone in having scleroderma or even in having a chronic disease. In fact, it is estimated that more than 50 million Americans suffer from some type of chronic illness. Knowing that others are suffering from a similar condition will not lessen the pain and loneliness you're feeling right now; that will happen over time. You may even feel as though you've been singled out. My friend Cheryl did. She was in a constant state of "Why me?" for several months. It wasn't until she joined a support group that she really believed she wasn't alone. But you have to do what feels right to you. Facts and figures won't make you feel less alone. You yourself have to do that. In time, as you learn more about scleroderma, you will begin to feel more comfortable with your diagnosis and less alone with your disease.

It's not your fault. As you learned in Day 1, getting scleroderma is not your fault. You didn't do anything to cause your disease. Somehow, it seems easier if we can find something or someone to blame for getting a disease. But you can't in this case, so don't blame yourself. Blame only causes guilt. And, God knows, you don't need another emotion to deal with right now. I know firsthand how emotionally devastating it can be to not know the cause of your disease. I felt the same way. But stop questioning yourself. You didn't do anything wrong. Leave it to the scientists to figure out.

Your life will change. Like it or not, your life will be different from this point forward. Not that that's necessarily a bad thing. But like most people, you're probably resistant to change. And you're probably feeling that you're ill-prepared to deal with the adaptations and adjustments your new disease is dictating. Some of the changes you may experience will be minor—such as needing to get more rest, or having to change your diet. Other changes are more profound—such as loss of a job. The key to successfully managing your life with a chronic disease is not in how many changes you have to make but in how well you accept and adapt to the changes.

There is no cure. I know this sounds scary, but keep in mind there are hundreds of diseases without cures. This doesn't mean you're going to die. Scleroderma's symptoms are treatable. You just have to find the right treatment for you. But it may take some time. In the meantime, take a deep breath and try to relax.

Life goes on. Fortunately, life doesn't stop just because you were diagnosed with scleroderma. Some days, though, you may feel like it should. People still need to go to work, go to school, and take care of families. You do, too. Your life is just different now. But it will go on. Take as much time as you need in accepting your life with a chronic disease. People do it every day. You can, too.

Your disease is in good company

As you also learned in Day 1, scleroderma is classified as an autoimmune disease. According to the American Autoimmune Related Diseases Association (AARDA), the term *autoimmune disease* refers to a

Common Autoimmune Diseases

HERE is a list of some of the more common autoimmune diseases you may be familiar with:

DISEASE	DISEASE TARGET
Multiple sclerosis	The myelin sheath surrounding the nerves in the brain and the spinal cord
Lupus	The joints, skin, kidneys, lungs, blood vessels, and brain
Rheumatoid arthritis	Membranes lining the joints
Sjögren's syndrome	The moisture-producing glands in the mouth, eyes, and vagina
Type 1 diabetes	Insulin-producing cells in the pancreas

group of more than 80 chronic illnesses, which involve almost every organ system. They can run from the very mild to the severe. For reasons unknown, about 75 percent of autoimmune diseases occur in women, most frequently during their childbearing years. These diseases are among the most poorly understood of any category of illnesses. Statistics from the AARDA show that autoimmune diseases are the fifth leading cause of death among women 15 to 44, separate from accidents, homicides, and suicides. This is not meant to scare you. In fact, it sheds great light on just how far we need to go in the search for causes and cures.

How common is scleroderma?

As you read earlier, it is estimated that there are 300,000 people diagnosed with scleroderma in the United States. Those figures jump to an estimated 700,000 when you include those diagnosed with scleroderma-like disorders. Scleroderma-like disorders resemble scleroderma but have their own distinct features. These related disorders include **eosinophilic fasciitis, scleromyxedema, chronic graft versus host disease**, and **eosinophilia myalgia syndrome**.

There is no definitive answer as to whether scleroderma is more common now than in the past. However, there seem to be more cases now than ever before. One reason for the apparent increase may be that some doctors have become more educated on scleroderma as well as more savvy in diagnosing the disease. I know this may seem hard to believe for those of you who had to go through a lengthy diagnostic process. There's no doubt that scleroderma is a difficult disease to diagnose. But scleroderma is becoming more widely known, thanks to the PR efforts of local and national scleroderma organizations. And don't forget the patients themselves. They have made tremendous strides in educating themselves and in getting the word out about scleroderma. And the benefits are long-lasting. The more PR the disease gets, the better the chances for more government funding to find a cure. So tell a friend who will tell another friend, and so on, and so on.

IN A SENTENCE:

> *Learning some basic information about scleroderma will help you to feel more in control of your disease.*

learning

The Many Faces of Scleroderma

THE GOOD news is, you finally have a diagnosis. The bad news is you've just been diagnosed with a very complicated disease. In Day 1, you learned about what type of disease scleroderma is. In this chapter, you'll learn about the many types of scleroderma. And because of the many directions the disease can take, you may feel as though you need a road map to truly understand what you're dealing with. You're not alone. Even doctors get confused about the types and the terminology. If you already know what type of scleroderma you have, it may be easier for you just to read that particular section right now. You can always come back later to learn more about the other types when you're not feeling so overwhelmed. If you're unsure about which type you have, or if whether your type has yet to be defined, rest assured I'm a pretty good navigator; I promise to keep you on the right track.

An overview

Scleroderma (often called systemic sclerosis in textbooks) is divided into two main categories:

1. *Localized scleroderma*—This form usually affects only the skin and does not involve internal organs.
2. *Systemic scleroderma*—This form typically involves both the skin and the internal organs.

Within each of these categories are subgroups. So now the disease looks like this:

1. *Localized scleroderma*
   - ○ Morphea
   - ○ Linear
   - ○ En coup de sabre (some consider this to be part of linear scleroderma)
2. *Systemic scleroderma*
   - ○ Limited (often referred to as CREST)
   - ○ Diffuse
   - ○ Scleroderma sine sclerosis

Breaking it down

Now comes the hard part. Although each subgroup has a specific definition of what it involves, keep in mind that there are always exceptions to the rules. So if you read something here that may be different from what you've experienced, don't get alarmed. As you learn more about your new disease, you'll soon realize there's nothing typical about scleroderma.

The *localized* form of scleroderma consists of the following:

○ **Morphea**—This is the most common form of localized scleroderma and refers to patches of thickened skin with varying degrees of pigment changes. The patches are typically oval and can vary in size and color. Although most commonly appearing on the trunk, the patches can appear anywhere on the body. Morphea has its own subtypes (not to be confused with the scleroderma subgroups):

1. *Localized morphea*—In this group, most patients develop only a few patches, which can evolve gradually over a period of months or years.

2. *Generalized morphea*—In this group, much more of the skin is involved. The patches can be so extensive they join together, involving most of the body surface.

Although no treatment has been proven to alter the course of **morphea scleroderma**, some patients do respond to certain ointments and medications. In localized morphea, the skin often improves within two to three years.

○ **Linear**—This type of scleroderma is more common in children and adolescents. Unlike morphea, **linear scleroderma** involves a band or line of thickened skin, which usually extends down an arm or a leg. And while morphea only affects the skin and fatty tissue under the skin surface, linear can also affect the underlying muscle and bone. If the line of thickened skin covers a joint, it can limit the motion of the joint. Efforts must be made to maintain full motion of the affected joint to avoid permanent damage. The phases of linear scleroderma are the same as in morphea. Typically, the disease will go through an active stage and, once stabilized, go through a recovery phase in which the thickened skin returns to a normal texture. Unfortunately, the underlying tissue of the thickened skin doesn't always return to normal and can cause some subtle changes in appearance.
○ **En coup de sabre**—This form of localized scleroderma is potentially the most disfiguring and occurs when linear scleroderma involves the head. Oftentimes, **en coup de sabre** begins on the forehead and spreads to involve the entire face. It can cause many different types of problems, including hair loss, unsightly indentations, and loss of fatty tissue under the skin.

Localized scleroderma often improves on its own over time, but the damage that occurs when the disease is active can be permanent. And because this type of scleroderma is more common in children than in adults, patients must work very closely with their physicians to make sure that their quality of life isn't adversely affected.

The *systemic* form of scleroderma consists of the following:

○ **Limited**—This type of scleroderma is often referred to as the **CREST** form. CREST is an acronym that stands for:

○ **C**alcinosis: Calcium deposits in the soft tissue of the skin.

○ **R**aynaud's phenomenon: Most commonly seen in the hands, this is a condition in which the small blood vessels contract in response to cold or anxiety. The fingertips usually turn white, blue, and/or red and often become numb.

○ **E**sophageal dysfunction: This refers to impaired function of the esophagus, often including swallowing difficulties and chronic heartburn.

○ **S**clerodactyly: This means thick and tight skin on the fingers due to excess collagen. The fingers are often difficult to bend or straighten.

○ **T**elangiectasias: Most commonly found on the face and hands, telangiectasias are small red spots caused by the dilation of blood vessels in the skin. Although not harmful, they can often create cosmetic problems for those affected by them.

The terms *CREST* and *limited scleroderma* are often used interchangeably. And you don't have to have all five of the above symptoms to be diagnosed with CREST. The main difference between limited and diffuse is the extent of the skin involvement as well as the onset of disease. Both forms include internal organ involvement, but limited scleroderma tends to come on more gradually and typically affects the skin on the face, fingers, hands, lower arms, and legs.

○ **Diffuse**—Although patients' experiences with diffuse scleroderma may vary, typically the onset of the disease is much more rapid than in limited (CREST). Skin thickening occurs more rapidly and includes more areas of the body, such as the trunk, hands, upper arms and legs, and the face. The patient usually feels quite ill and sometimes experiences loss of appetite, extreme fatigue, as well as joint aches and pain. Because of the potential damage to the heart, lungs, kidneys, and GI tract, early diagnosis and continual monitoring are crucial in diffuse scleroderma.

○ **Scleroderma sine sclerosis**—This type of scleroderma resembles either limited or diffuse scleroderma, including the organ involvement typically seen in both types. However, the main difference is that this type of scleroderma does not affect the skin.

Take your time in digesting this

Although all this information seems like a lot to swallow at once, keep in mind this is for reference purposes only. Your goal right now should be to focus on your particular type of scleroderma. If your type has yet to be diagnosed, be patient. This is completely normal. Localized scleroderma is more easily recognized and diagnosed due to the overt skin changes; systemic tends to be a bit harder to diagnose, especially in the beginning.

IN A SENTENCE:

> *Scleroderma is a very complicated disease, involving many different types and scenarios.*

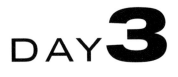

DAY **3**

living

Managing Your Disease— What's Your Style?

YOU'VE HAD a few days to deal with your diagnosis and you're still a wreck. Only now, you realize you have a much greater task ahead of you: managing your disease.

Ostrich or lion?

Sheri, upon learning of her diagnosis, became an ostrich. She stuck her head in the sand. She didn't want to know a thing about her disease. And when Sheri found out that her mom went to a scleroderma support meeting to learn more about the disease, she was mortified. Sheri didn't want to admit that there was anything wrong with her. Not to herself and not to others. Hers was a classic case of denial. It took her years to accept her disease.

I, on the other hand, was a lion, with a voracious appetite for information. I couldn't get enough. I wanted to know what I was in for and I wanted to know immediately. I tried to walk myself through as many possible scenarios as I could, to prepare myself for what might possibly happen to me. I'd go to my doctors armed with lists of questions, half of which they couldn't answer. So I'd look elsewhere for the answers and try to sift through the mountains of misinformation I came across. Overkill? Perhaps. But it worked for me. Through my research, I felt more capable of making informed decisions about my treatment and care.

These two examples are rather extreme; your management style probably lies somewhere in between. There is no right or wrong style. You must manage your disease in the way that feels right for you. And your initial reaction to your disease may or may not be indicative of how you ultimately choose to manage your disease. But if you find your reactions are ruling your actions, you've found your management style. Keep in mind that each management style has its advantages and disadvantages. But however we choose to cope, we must all come to terms with our disease and manage it the best way we know how.

What's your style?

Are you a control freak? Or do new situations paralyze you? Maybe denial's your thing. Or perhaps, indifference. Yours may even be a combination of styles. That's okay, too. But remember, whatever your style is, your goal is to get to a place of acceptance and control. For some, that's not such an easy path—particularly if their management style does not allow acceptance and control to come about naturally. Over the years, I've learned not to judge people by how they manage their disease just because their style is different from mine. Everybody's different. If your way of handling things sounds crazy to those around you, so be it. You know what your goal is. Give yourself time and you'll get there, too.

The elephant theory: recognize your style?

Have you ever heard the anecdote about having something huge and important going on in your life that's happening right under your nose but you choose to ignore its presence? It's sometimes referred to as "the elephant in the room." Imagine your disease is the elephant. And the elephant is sitting in the middle of the room. When you walk into the room, how do you approach the elephant? Many different scenarios come to mind, and they all represent different management styles. Which one is yours?

1. **Denial.** You enter the room and everybody is talking about the elephant. You say to yourself, "What elephant? I don't see it. It wasn't there before, therefore it doesn't exist." Yep, you know where I'm going with this. Sometimes the truth is too hard too handle and you don't want to see what's right in front of you. Denying the fact that you have scleroderma may be the only way you are able to deal with it right now. It's a very normal reaction. Eventually, though, you'll have to come to terms with it. You can't manage a disease when you're in denial. Your health and well-being are dependent on your acceptance of scleroderma. It doesn't have to happen today, or even tomorrow. But it does have to happen. You deserve the best care and treatment, and acknowledging you have a disease will allow you to get it.

2. **Fear.** After walking into the room, you take one look at the elephant and run out, screaming at the top of your lungs. It's called fear. And fear can emotionally paralyze you. Being diagnosed with scleroderma certainly can be very frightening. That fear can overrule every other emotion you're feeling. But don't let your fear stop you from acknowledging your health problems. This only leads to major problems down the road. Early intervention is crucial in a disease like scleroderma. You'll learn more about this in Week 2. Break it down into baby steps. Open the door to the room just a little bit each day. Eventually, you'll be able to walk into the room and stand right by the elephant's side. But do take your time. Elephants are large animals.

3. **Indifference.** You open the door to the room, look at the elephant, acknowledge it, and lazily walk back out the door. It doesn't seem to have an effect on you one way or another. The good news is you won't be focusing on the negative aspects of the disease, but that's also the bad news: You won't be focusing on *anything* about the disease. Often, new symptoms arise that require your immediate attention. It's great not to be too overwhelmed with your disease. But you can't neglect it, either. You need to be able to jump into action when the need arises.

4. **Acceptance.** As soon as you see the elephant, you go right up to it, pet it, and give it a big hug. Then you climb on top of it. Afterward, you move some furniture around and rearrange the room to accommodate the elephant. This new room arrangement makes the elephant look like it belongs. This does not mean you love having a new

disease. Nor does it mean it belongs. It simply means you've accepted the cards you've been dealt and have incorporated your disease into your lifestyle. This is a very practical way to manage your disease. Your life will become much easier because of it.

5. **Anger.** Your first impulse upon seeing the elephant is to hurt it. Don't. You'll only be hurting yourself. It's normal to feel angry in the beginning. But then, let it go. Anger makes you bitter—and causes you a lot of stress. Scleroderma and stress are a lethal combination. Do whatever you can to help yourself feel less angry: See a therapist, throw pillows, run around the block—you get the idea. It's hard to manage a disease when you feel angry all the time. It just gets in the way.

6. **Control freak.** As soon as you see the elephant, you want to know everything there is to know about him: where he was born, how much he weighs, how tall he is, and so on. Your need to learn about this strange new creature is unrelenting. You'll do anything to feel like you have some control over it. It's fabulous to want to know exactly what you're dealing with. Just realize you may not get all the answers all the time. And some of the answers you get, you may not like.

7. **Intimidation.** At first sight of the animal, you feel small and unworthy. When he moves, you move to accommodate him. When he walks out the door, you follow. When he turns around, you turn around, too. You're constantly trying to please the elephant—you don't want to upset it. Stop. Don't be a doormat. Don't give all the control to the animal. Sure, he's big. Sure, he takes up a lot of space. But remember, you're the boss. The elephant is just as scared of you as you are of him. Don't let your disease manage you. You manage your disease . . . as best you can.

8. **Attention seeker.** The elephant in the room makes you feel special when you're around it. You like the extra attention it brings you. In fact, it may be just the kind of attention you've been seeking. And it feels nice to finally have it. It's great to be the center of attention if you just got a new hairstyle, or maybe even a promotion at work. But you didn't. You just found out you have a serious disease. Don't use it as an accessory for others to focus on. You will begin to resent it the minute you don't get the results you're after. You have a disease, not a new haircut. Try to manage it accordingly.

Obviously, your management style in the first few days of your diagnosis may not be indicative of how you ultimately handle things. You may even be feeling numb right now. This is your life and disease. You need to manage it in the way that feels most comfortable to you. Don't try to fit into any management style that is not right for you or for the way you handle things. Remember, you're in charge. But you need to be aware of how your management style impacts the decisions you need to make in your day-to-day management of scleroderma. Your health and well-being depend on it.

IN A SENTENCE:

> *There are many different ways to manage your disease; just make sure your management style doesn't do you more harm than good.*

learning

Friends and Family:
What to Expect ... or Not

I KNOW you know this, but I'm going to say it anyway. Not everyone in your life is going to react to your news the way you expect they will. Their reactions will range from shock to anger to pity to support to sympathy, etc. In fact, the reactions of those around you will probably be quite similar to some of the feelings you had upon hearing your diagnosis. But here's the tricky part. You don't know who in your life is going to have which reaction. I was constantly surprised by people's reactions when I told them about my new disease. Some of those who I thought were going to be the least supportive ended up being the most supportive. And on the opposite end, some of the people whom I expected would be there for me virtually disappeared. I finally learned not to have any expectations from those I told. This way, I was never too surprised or disappointed by their reaction to my news. You, too, will probably be both surprised and humbled by many in your life. So prepare yourself for some unpredictable reactions.

Know your audience

At this point, the most logical thing to talk about would be how to break the news about your disease to your spouse, your child, your boss, your parents, your teacher, or whomever. But I don't know your friends or your family, and I'm certainly not qualified to tell you whom you should or shouldn't tell. That's up to you. What I will tell you is, know your audience. Try to think about what you know about this person and how he or she reacts in certain situations. Does the person become very emotional? Is the person self-absorbed? Does he or she worry excessively? Is he or she sympathetic? Your answers to these questions will determine how much information you want to reveal and how the person is likely to react to your news.

For example, say you have someone in your life who is a constant worrier, and you know that no matter what you say about your disease, the person will worry about every detail you relate. In this instance, it's better to filter the amount of information you deliver; save the gorier details for someone better equipped to handle them. Be honest, be forthcoming, but don't overwhelm the worrier with information that may be too hard to digest.

As for me, I was constantly surprised—often happily—by the reactions of those I told. One time, during a particularly difficult period, an acquaintance of mine from my children's school not only cooked dinner for my entire family but also offered to take my kids to school for the rest of the week. I will never forget the kindness showered upon my family and me from someone I had not expected it from.

There is no typical response you can expect when telling people about your disease. As much as you hope the person you tell will react in a kind, loving, and supportive manner, unfortunately, that won't always be the case.

The different types of responses you may receive

Friends and family come in all shapes and forms and will respond to your news in just as many ways. Rather than telling you whom you should tell and how, I'll share with you some of the many different types of responses you may get; then you can work backward and fill in the blanks of who in your life might respond that way. I'm sure you will recognize many of your loved ones within this list.

○ The *"I can't handle your news"* response: The number of people in your life with this response is probably more than you would like. Especially if they're close to you. Many people, understandably, don't handle the news of a loved one's ill health very well. Some go into denial. Some need more time to adjust to the news. Some just don't want to hear it. The best thing you can do is be patient with them. Don't give them lots of information at once. Spoonfeed the details to them and stay calm. In time, they will become more comfortable with your disease, once they are more familiar with what you're dealing with and how you're affected by it.

○ The *"I don't want to hear the details; just the facts, please"* response: Some people in your life are there to give you support and others are there to offer advice. And some are there to just listen. Don't expect this group to offer support. They're not interested in hearing about the day-to-day trials of living with a chronic disease. They want information, not details. Your boss may be a good example of this type of person, wanting only to hear the bottom line. The other stuff just gets in the way.

○ The *"Oh, I'm so sorry, but let me tell you about my trip to Tahiti"* response: Don't bother giving these people any more information. And certainly don't look to them for understanding. These people are self-absorbed, period.

○ The *"What can I do to help you"* response: Thank your lucky stars for this group. These people will stick with you through thick and thin. You can lean on them for both support and advice. And they're good listeners. These people truly want to help you and be there for you. They'll babysit your kids, go to the market for you, drive you to your appointments, and so on. Try to surround yourself with this type of warmth and generosity. These people are exactly whom you need in your life right now.

○ The *"Why didn't you ask the doctor this question"* or, *"You shouldn't have agreed to take that test so soon"* response: This group tends to be very judgmental. Instead of just listening to you, they judge your every move. It's hard enough to make decisions about your health every day, let alone feel like you're being judged on the choices you make. You're in a very vulnerable place. You need to feel that you're being supported, not judged. Think twice before sharing information with this group next time. You don't need to be feeling judged, particularly now.

○ The *"Here's what I think you ought to do"* response: Instead of just listening to you, this group wants to tell you what to do. If you ask for advice, that's one thing. But if the advice comes unsolicited, that's another matter. Such people tend to be problem-solvers and feel they are being helpful by offering solutions to your problems. I would think twice about giving them many details if you're not looking for advice, because you're going to get some whether you like it or not.

○ The *"I can't believe you're canceling plans, again"* response: These people are not your friends. They certainly don't have your best interests at heart. And they couldn't possibly care about how you're feeling. Drop them. Fast.

○ The *"I want to hear every detail"* response: Sometimes you feel like sharing a lot of details. Other times, you don't. These people tend to be draining. Give them only what you feel comfortable disclosing. Nothing more, nothing less.

○ The *"I'd love to be there for you, but I'm so busy right now. I'll call you soon"* response: These people may truly be well-intentioned but are incapable of being there for you. Perhaps emotionally, they can't handle your news. Don't expect them to stick around. They may check in with you now and then, but that's about it. You may feel very let down by people with this response. Try not to have any expectations about them. You will surely be setting yourself up for disappointment. Try, instead, to move forward without them. Maybe one day, in the future, they will come around again, when they feel better equipped emotionally to deal with your needs.

○ The *"But how am I supposed to deal with this"* response: This group may truly be devastated by your news. And they're very worried about how this news is going to affect them. But be careful. They may be looking to you to take care of their feelings. Resist the urge to jump in. You've got enough on your own plate. Let them find support for their own feelings from others besides yourself. Forgive them for being needy right now. They need time to adjust to the news, too.

○ The *"Please get in bed right now, get plenty of rest, don't overdo it, etc."* response: These people have big hearts and care deeply about you. You might get this type of response from a parent or a spouse. They want to protect you and take care of you. Just make sure they don't smother you. Let them do for you only what you're comfortable with, and make sure they know you're still capable of making your own choices and decisions. It feels great to be taken care of. But don't lose yourself in the process.

Remember, it is up to you to decide whom you should tell and how much you want to disclose. There are no rules to this. You're in charge. In the beginning, you may decide not to tell a certain person, only to decide later you would like to share the news. That's okay. And if you don't feel like telling anyone, that's okay, too. Ultimately, you are only responsible to yourself for the choices you make. These are your feelings and your choices. Follow your instincts.

IN A SENTENCE:

> *Only you can decide how much or how little you want to reveal and to whom you want to reveal it.*

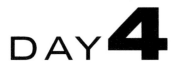

DAY **4**

living

What Am I
Going to Look Like?

IT'S BAD enough to be diagnosed with a rare, incurable, chronic disease. But it's adding insult to injury to have to worry about how the disease is going to change your looks. Although many changes can occur, thickened skin is the most noticeable feature of the disease. And although some forms of scleroderma don't affect your skin (**scleroderma sine sclerosis**), most forms do. The changes may be limited to the fingers (**sclero-dactyly**) or may involve the backs of the hands, the forearms, upper arms, trunk, legs, and feet. Scleroderma can also affect the skin on the face. Typically, the skin thickening reaches its maximum scope within three to five years after onset, then begins to soften again.

The hands and face

Some areas of the body affected by scleroderma are easily concealed; other parts, such as your hands and face, are nearly impossible to hide. When I asked some patients what their biggest concerns were about the physical changes caused by scleroderma, most said they were fearful about how the disease would change their looks; loss of function came in a close second. Here are some of their reactions:

○ When Christie was first diagnosed, she saw a picture of another patient's hands and face and burst into tears. She was just beginning to model and was terrified about what was going to happen to her and what she might look like.

○ After Maria was diagnosed, she was fearful of looking disfigured.

○ Shirley was so ashamed of how her hands looked, she often kept them in her pockets or kept her sleeves rolled all the way down to cover them.

○ Lydia's biggest fear was what her face was going to look like. She said, "I know it sounds so vain, but I have to admit that not knowing what I'd turn into was the scariest thing for me. I was watching my hands and face change day by day. Secondary to how I was going to look, my biggest fear was not being able to care for myself."

Sound familiar? Many illnesses involve disease- and/or treatment-related changes in appearance; however, very few researchers have studied these. One study, however, assessed how scleroderma patients felt about their appearance. In the 1999 study published in *Cognitive Therapy and Research*, 93 people received clinical examinations of their skin thickening. In addition, each patient completed a questionnaire about their appearance self-esteem and their overall psychological distress. The results found that those patients who had lower self-esteem about their physical appearance reported the greatest amount of psychological distress. One of the study's most interesting findings was that one of the best predictors of distress from the physical changes was seen in those patients who had skin thickening of the right hand and fingers. Because the right hand is usually dominant, this finding seems to make logical sense. You'll read more about hand changes a little later in the chapter.

Scleroderma-related facial changes

Both physical and functional facial changes can occur as a result of scleroderma. Currently, there is no available data regarding the exact number of patients affected by facial changes. However, these changes are a real possibility for most individuals with the systemic as well as the localized form of the disease, although to a much lesser extent. We'll talk more about the physical limitations in the Learning section of this chapter. As is the case with just about everything that happens in scleroderma, facial changes can vary greatly from patient to patient. They can occur over a period of a few months up to several years. The most common facial changes include

○ loss of facial mobility and expression
○ **microstomia** (small mouth)
○ difficulty in opening the mouth wide—which can impair eating, brushing, flossing, and dental care abilities
○ loss of mobility in the upper lip—making it difficult to close the mouth as well as chew food
○ extreme tightness in the facial muscles
○ **telangiectasias** (red spots caused by the dilatation of small blood vessels in the skin)

Keep in mind that very few patients are affected by everything listed above. And this list is only of the most common facial changes that can happen. If you're experiencing any new symptoms or changes such as the ones listed above, remember to discuss them with your physician.

Often, these changes can cause a loss of facial expression and skills which in turn can lead to a loss of identity. Loss of identity can be one of the most devastating aspects of the disease. But remember: Underneath it all, you're still you. Just because you look different doesn't mean you are different. Never forget that who you are on the inside is not based on what you look like on the outside.

Another form of scleroderma that can affect the face is a localized form called en coup de sabre. A French term meaning "cut of the sword," this form of scleroderma was named because the scarring resembles a saber wound. This type of scleroderma usually begins as an indentation on the forehead or at the frontal hairline. The line of the thickened skin may spread to involve the entire face but is usually confined to only one side and does not involve the body. There also may be loss of the fatty tissue on the affected side of the face. Unfortunately, little research has been done on successfully treating this form of linear scleroderma.

Scleroderma hand changes

Diffuse swelling throughout the hands is often one of the first symptoms of scleroderma. Patients have often described their fingers as "sausage-like" in this early phase of the disease. Once this phase is over, the skin on the fingers and hands begins to tighten, causing the fingers to curl inward. And sometimes the tightened skin may cause **contractures**. A contracture means that the joint cannot be fully flexed or extended. Maintaining motion in these joints may require daily exercises to ensure your hands retain as much mobility as possible. Unfortunately, contractures can also cause the hands to look deformed.

Another problem that can occur with the hands are skin **ulcers**. And they are much more than just a cosmetic problem. Caused by poor circulation, "digital ulcers" can be extremely painful and can interfere with function. If this a problem for you, please speak with your physician about the best treatment options. Losing the ability to use your hands often means having to reassess everything from your hobbies, to the kind of work you do, to your home environment.

Other skin problems that can occur

- ○ *Itching*: Early on in systemic scleroderma, some people may experience severe itching in the involved skin.
- ○ *Dryness*: As skin changes occur, the skin's ability to sweat often becomes impaired, causing dry skin.
- ○ *Calcium deposits* (**calcinosis**): Calcium salts may accumulate under the skin in the soft tissue; they'll feel like bumps under the skin. They are often painful when pressure is applied and can become especially troublesome if located on pressure sites such as the fingertips, elbows, or knees.

As with all aspects of scleroderma, you may or may not be affected by any of the above physical manifestations of the disease. If you are, you'll learn more about how to cope with these physical changes in the Learning section of this chapter. Being aware of some of these physical changes is the first step to recognizing and dealing with a very real aspect of the disease, which often gets swept under the rug. Once you acknowledge your limitations, you can begin to work toward accepting these changes. And knowing you're not alone can often make all the difference in how you cope.

IN A SENTENCE:

> *The physical manifestations of scleroderma, especially to the hands and face, can be devastating—but acknowledgment is the first step toward acceptance.*

learning

Dealing with the Physical Changes

THE PERSONAL and social impact of scleroderma-related physical changes is enormous. As you learned in the Living section of this chapter, some patients are more concerned with how the disease is going to affect the way they look, while others are more concerned with remaining functional. But no matter what your concerns are, the changes that occur can have a tremendous impact on your self-esteem, leading to feelings of anxiety and isolation. Emotionally, this may be one of the most difficult aspects of the disease. Before we address how to cope with these changes, let's take a look at a study on body image among women with scleroderma and its relationship to psychosocial function.

Body-image dissatisfaction

In a 2003 study published in *Health Psychology*, body-image dissatisfaction and its relationship to psychosocial function was investigated in 127 women with scleroderma. Surprisingly, the results indicated that body-image dissatisfaction for this group of women was higher than that of a sample of patients with severe burn injuries. And although the results suggest that younger patients with more severe disease may be at greatest risk for developing body-image concerns, most of the women in the study felt very strong dissatisfaction about the physical changes caused by the disease. Early identification and treatment of body-image dissatisfaction may help prevent the development of both depression and psychosocial impairment and should be assessed routinely.

If your physician has never discussed with you the many physical changes that can occur in scleroderma, they can be particularly devastating. Part of your ability to cope with these changes depends on knowing what to expect.

Acknowledging your fears

Scleroderma patients speak out about their fears and how they dealt with them:

○ When Bonnie H. was first diagnosed, her biggest fear was about dying. But as soon as her hands began to curl and her feet became stiff, she was more afraid of not being functional. She dealt with the physical changes by "distancing her brain from her body."

○ At first, Bonnie D. was more annoyed than fearful about what was happening to her hands. But when her hands began to hurt, she became very fearful of the pain. Her solution was to get adaptive aids like rubber door handles for her doors and rubber knobs for the light switches.

○ Josephine was much more frightened of the physical limitations the disease causes than of how she was going to look. She went to physical therapy and used putty to help exercise her hands.

Learning to cope

One of the first steps in coping with scleroderma's physical changes is acknowledgment. You have experienced a loss, whether it be physical or functional, and you must allow yourself time to grieve. Once you have acknowledged your loss, it's time to take some action. Consider any of the following strategies:

1. *Talk to a mental health professional.* Our society places an enormous value on health and beauty. A loss in this area wreaks havoc on your self-esteem. You might begin to avoid social situations, which will only increase your sense of isolation. Stop the cycle by confronting your fears and getting help. If you're not comfortable speaking to a therapist, find someone else: a family member, a close friend, another patient, or perhaps a coworker.

2. *Join a support group.* You may feel as if you're the only one who's had to experience these awful changes and that no one understands what you're going through. Not true. Joining a support group not only allows you to actually see others with the same physical changes as you, but also allows you to share feelings and experiences. You are not alone. And don't feel as if you need to experience these changes on your own, either.

3. *Make sure your pain is controlled.* Pain can be both physically and emotionally draining. Consult your medical team about trying to minimize or eliminate your pain. If that doesn't work, see a pain specialist. Ask your rheumatologist for a referral.

4. *Work with a physical or occupational therapist.* Maintaining mobilty and remaining functional are big concerns for some patients. You may want to work with an occupational therapist to develop a plan for maintaining motion in your hands and face.

5. *Treat your skin problems as best you can:*

   - ○ **Dryness:** Avoid excessive bathing and handwashing. Use lotions high in lanolin, such as: Vaseline Intensive Care, Nivea, and Neutrogena Norwegian Formula. Also use vitamin E–based skin care products like Alpha Keri lotion and bath oils. They should be applied several times a day, particularly after you've been in water.
   - ○ **Itching:** Try using oatmeal-based cleanser bars like Aveeno. Topical steroids may be used, as well as **antipruitics** (anti-itching meds). The itching will undoubtedly decrease later in the disease and its stopping is often a good prognostic sign.
   - ○ **Ulcerations and calcinosis:** Both manifestations can become quite complicated and require ongoing treatment from a knowledgeable physician.

In a society that places so much value on beauty and looks, the physical manifestations of scleroderma are often the most devastating. Your coping skills in this area rely on acceptance of your physical limitations. There are lots of ways to deal with these issues—just make sure you work closely with your physician to ensure the most promising results.

IN A SENTENCE:

> *Learning to cope with the physical manifestations of scleroderma can often be the biggest challenge—but there's plenty of help, emotional and physical, if you need it.*

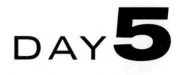

Get a Good Quarterback

FINDING A doctor to treat your disease sounds like a pretty easy thing to do. And often, it is. But let's stop and think for a minute. Remember what you went through to get a diagnosis? Seeing doctor after doctor after doctor? Enough said. Perhaps you were diagnosed by a savvy PCP (primary care physician) or a dermatologist. Kudos to that person for knowing enough about the disease to give you a diagnosis. Now it's time to look at the bigger picture. You deserve the best care and treatment to help you manage the disease that you now, finally, have a name for. Enter the almighty rheumatologist.

The rheumatologist

According to the American College of Rheumatology, a rheumatologist is an internist or pediatrician who is qualified by additional training and experience in the diagnosis and treatment of arthritis and other diseases of the joints, muscles, and bones. A rheumatologist's credentials include four years of medical school followed by three years of training and an additional two to three years in specialized rheumatology training. Rheumatologists treat more than 100 types of diseases, including scleroderma, rheumatoid arthritis, lupus, and osteoarthritis.

Because of the complexity of many rheumatic diseases, it takes time to develop the right course of treatment; moveover, these types of diseases often evolve over time.

In many situations, the rheumatologist acts as a "quarterback" for your medical team. You'll learn more about the importance of teamwork in the Learning section of this chapter.

What to look for

In a sentence, All doctors are not created equal. And even doctors within the same specialty are not created equal. Although rheumatologists treat all types of rheumatic disease, many develop an expertise in one particular type of disease. Your goal is to find a rheumatologist who is an expert in treating scleroderma. Picking the right one is crucial to your well-being. How much time do you spend shopping for something far less significant than your health—like new furniture or a car? You probably spend more time shopping for these things than you'd like to admit. Now you're shopping for something far more important: your health for the rest of your life. The doctor you choose probably will be in your life for years to come. Take your time and choose wisely.

There are several things to consider when beginning your search:

1. **What are your needs as a patient?** Do you like to be told what to do or would you prefer to be involved in the decision-making process? Determining your own style will help you choose what style to look for in a physician. If you like to be told what to do and have no desire to be involved in the decisions regarding your treatment and care, you need to look for an authoritarian physician. This type of doctor will be more than happy to tell you what to do. And believe me, there are plenty out there to choose from. But if you'd like to be involved in the decision-making process (which I strongly encourage), you need to look for a physician who won't feel threatened by your questions and input. When Isabel told her doctor she didn't like the treatment he recommended, he told her to look for a different doctor. Obviously, this is not the type of physician you want when you're an involved, proactive patient. Make sure the rheumatologist you choose is will-

ing to listen to your input and is respectful of your need to have some
sense of control over your situation.

2. **How long has the physician been in practice?** Remember, it's
   all a numbers game. The longer they've been in practice, the more
   patients they've seen. Longevity equals experience. Experience is
   crucial when dealing with a disease like scleroderma.

3. **Is the physician associated with a well-known hospital?** And,
   is the hospital geographically convenient for you and your relatives?
   Try to think ahead as much as possible. This may never apply to you,
   but, on the off chance that you'll need to be hospitalized during the
   course of your disease, you need to think about the hospital your
   physician is associated with. A few things to consider:

   ○ Is the hospital near you and your relatives? Hospitals are lonely
   places, if you don't have a familiar face to cheer you up. Make
   sure it's accessible to you and those around you.

   ○ Is the hospital on your insurance plan? This important detail is
   often overlooked. I almost became a victim of the system when the
   hospital of my choice decided to not renew their contract with my
   insurance company. Luckily, they were finally able to come to an
   agreement after several months . . . but not without lots of anxiety-
   filled months, for me.

4. **How many of the physician's patients are scleroderma
   patients?** Again, the more scleroderma patients the physician has
   seen, the more knowledgeable he or she is in treating you. If the doctor claims to be a scleroderma expert but has only treated a handful
   of patients over the years, choose another physician.

5. **Is the physician involved in research and/or clinical trials?**
   This can be important if you're looking for the latest treatment
   options or would like to be involved in a clinical trial. The more up-
   to-date the physician is, the more he or she can offer you.

6. **Is the physician part of a large practice with multiple associ-
   ates, or a one-person show?** You never know when that strange
   new symptom will appear but oops, your doctor is away on a ski trip
   in Vail for three weeks. It's always nice to have backup from the same
   office.

7. **Is the office location geographically desirable?** Some people don't mind driving a long distance to their appointments; others do. Remember, you'll be having lots of follow-up appointments with your doctor. And some of those times, you may not be feeling so well. Make sure you're comfortable with the office location.

8. **Is the physician on your insurance plan?** Make sure you do your homework before you make your choice. Just as in choosing the hospital, when choosing a physician, this detail can be easily overlooked. Unfortunately, in today's society, this particular detail can often be the deal-breaker in your search.

One thing I learned along the way is that you don't always make the right choice on your first try . . . or even your second. The first rheumatologist I chose came with a fabulous recommendation, appropriate degrees on the walls, a friendly office staff, and a comfortable waiting room. What could go so wrong? It's called bedside manner. He turned out to be Godzilla in a white coat. He barked orders at me with a ferocity that scared the daylights out of me. I was horrified at his treatment of me as well as of his office staff. I knew instantly this was not the right doctor for me. So, I moved on to the next one.

The second physician I chose was just as disappointing as the first. My father nicknamed him "The Wizard of Oz." In the eight months that I was under his care, I think I only laid eyes on him twice. He was mysteriously absent for most of my appointments and virtually disappeared when I tried to reach him by phone. At one point, I even told the nurse I felt like Dorothy in search of the great Wizard. I was seen by resident after resident (this was a teaching hospital), because "the Wizard" was always being called away to something far more important than his patients. It seemed patient care was pretty low on his priority list. I often wondered why he had become a physician in the first place.

Now that you have a sense of what you might be looking for and how to go about finding it (see "Resources to help your search" on p.41), I'd like to point out a few additional considerations. The following issues are vital to insuring a successful relationship with your rheumatologist. You'll learn more about the importance of these issues in Month 2.

KEY ISSUES FOR A SUCCESSFUL DOCTOR-PATIENT RELATIONSHIP

○ Do you trust your physician?

○ Does he/she treat you with respect?

○ Is he/she a good listener?

○ Is he/she responsive to your phone calls?

○ Are you a good personality match?

○ Are you comfortable with his/her office staff?

○ Are you satisfied with his/her medical expertise?

If you've answered yes to the above questions, you've found your match. The key issue is, don't settle. If your first choice doesn't work out, you can always search again. Remember, you have a chronic disease and will have to spend quite a bit of time with your doctor. Make sure you're comfortable with the choice you've made. Never forget, you deserve the best treatment and care.

IN A SENTENCE:

Picking the right rheumatologist is essential to your long-term health and well-being.

learning

Assembling Your Medical Team

YOU'VE FINALLY found a rheumatologist; now you're wondering what other specialists you may need to see. For some of you, there may be an immediate need to build a medical team. Others of you may be able to wait a while. For most, it's an incredibly overwhelming process, mainly due to lack of experience. Who's ever had to put together a medical team before? And, just as in finding a rheumatologist, you might not make the right choices the first time around. I, for one, did not. It took me two years to put together my team. Now I couldn't be happier. But that was my experience. It doesn't have to be yours. The most important thing to remember while going through this process is, you are in charge. You'll go through plenty of times these first few weeks when you feel like you're not. So, stop and repeat: I am in charge.

What is a specialist?

According to the American Medical Association (AMA), a specialist concentrates on certain body systems, specific age groups, or complex scientific techniques developed to diagnose or treat certain types of disorders. Taking it a step further, a subspecialist is a physician who has completed training in a medical specialty and then takes additional training in a more specific area of that specialty (called a subspecialty). For example, rheumatology is a subspecialty of internal medicine. The training of a subspecialist within a specialty requires an additional one or more years of full-time education. You'll read more about the different types of specialists you may need later in this chapter.

Why you may need a specialist

At this point, your rheumatologist should have some idea of the severity of your disease. Perhaps he or she feels an organ is being threatened and that you need immediate intervention from a specialist. This is the time to trust your quarterback. Your rheumatologist will send you to a specialist he or she has worked with before and feels would best suit your needs. Get the consult first, and worry about how the specialist fits on your team later. This is the trial run. After you solve the medical crisis, then you can determine whether the consulting specialist is a first-rate choice. Keep in mind, you're looking for the same things you were looking for when finding a rheumatologist. Is the specialist competent? Does he or she listen to you? Are you a personality match? Does the physician respect you? Is he or she on your insurance plan? Also consider: Is the specialist a good fit with your rheumatologist? Don't ever underestimate the importance of this dynamic. Your rheumatologist will most likely be calling the shots. Make sure the doctors you choose are aware of this.

If there's no immediate medical crisis, you have time to actually do some homework. Here's how to get started.

HOW TO FIND A SPECIALIST AND WHAT TO LOOK FOR

○ *Ask your rheumatologist for recommendations.* Because of the nature of the disease, your rheumatologist has probably worked with virtually every type of specialist out there. The benefit to choosing a specialist with whom your doctor has worked is twofold:

1. The two doctors have already built a relationship by working together in the past. They know and trust each other and also respect each other's medical opinion.

2. The specialist your rheumatologist has chosen for you is probably very savvy on the complications of the disease. This is crucial. Just because a physician is a specialist doesn't mean he or she knows about all the complications of scleroderma.

○ ***Ask other scleroderma patients.*** When I was searching for a pulmonologist, I made the mistake of asking others who weren't scleroderma patients but who had basic pulmonary problems, like asthma or bronchitis. The physician who was recommended to me had a wonderful reputation and a lovely personality. Too bad he didn't know a thing about scleroderma. Remember, your goal is to not only find a fabulous specialist, but to find a fabulous specialist who is also an expert on scleroderma.

○ ***If possible, make sure all the specialists you choose are able to work out of the same hospital.*** Don't take for granted that they can. A physician has to have privileges at a specific hospital in order to work there. If you have one specialist who works at one end of town and another at the other end of town, they're most likely associated with different hospitals. Keep this in mind when choosing your medical team. If you are ever hospitalized, you'll need your physicians to be associated with the same hospital to be able to work together as a team, to give you the best care and treatment.

○ ***Call the Scleroderma Foundation.*** If you don't have a local chapter nearby, call the national office at 800-722-HOPE. The staff members will do their best to help you track down the specialist nearest you.

THE SPECIALISTS YOU'LL NEED ON YOUR TEAM

Your doctor has told you to see a kidney specialist. What type of doctor is that? Here's a list of the specialists you are most likely to need and what they do.

1. **Dermatologist:** A physician trained to diagnose and treat disorders of the skin, including recognition of the skin manifestations of systemic and infectious diseases

2. **Cardiologist:** An internist who specializes in diseases of the heart, lungs, and blood vessels

3. **Gastroenterologist:** An internist who specializes in diagnosis and treatment of the digestive organs, including the stomach, bowels, liver, and gallbladder
4. **Nephrologist (the kidney specialist mentioned above):** An internist who treats disorders of the kidneys, high blood pressure, fluid and mineral balance, and dialysis of body wastes when the kidneys do not function
5. **Pulmonologist:** An internist who treats disease of the lungs and airways

Your rheumatologist may also recommend that you see a physical therapist or an occupational therapist. The role of the physical therapist is to assist patients in achieving optimal function and pain relief; the role of the occupational therapist is to improve and maintain a patient's ability to perform activities of daily living that are functional and meaningful to that individual.

Most patients I know also have a mental health professional (psychologist, psychiatrist, or therapist) on their team. You may not need this person all the time, but it's nice to know the person is there for you when you need him or her.

Friction among the team members

Let's face it. Doctors are human. The white coat doesn't shield them from human emotion; they have feelings too. There will be times in the course of your disease when your doctors disagree—probably more often than you would like. But remember: You're part of the team too. Your opinion matters. (Have you been repeating, "I am in charge"?) As much as it might feel uncomfortable to you, you need to take an active role on the team. You have the right to make decisions about your health care. It's easy to forget this when you're not feeling well and just want to feel better. But don't lose sight of the fact that you have much more influence on your team than you think you have. Sometimes your feelings about a particular situation will help to resolve conflicts that have arisen among the team members. Your input, in essence, is invaluable to your team.

When conflicts arise among members of my medical team (and believe me, they do!), I listen to the differing opinions and then try to do some research on my own. I'm the one who has to live with whatever decision is made about my treatment and care. I would much prefer to be part of that decision-making process.

Your role on your medical team has to feel right to you. You might not feel as comfortable about jumping in when conflicts arise. That's okay. As time goes on, you'll find your comfort zone on your team. Your role is important. Just make sure it's an active one.

In the long run

Building your medical team can seem like a daunting task. If you can, take some time to do your homework and choose wisely. You'll find this pays off in the long run. And if you find you need a substitute player every now and then, that's okay, too. Hopefully, you won't need to see every type of specialist mentioned. Few people do. The good news: Now you are aware of both the terminology and the team-building process. You can move forward with confidence knowing you are able to build an excellent medical team if and when the time comes.

IN A SENTENCE:

> *The benefits of a medical team made up of scleroderma experts will result in better treatment and care for your disease.*

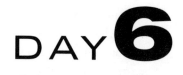

living

Raynaud's, Sjögren's, and Other Accompanying Conditions

YOU FINALLY have a name for your disease and are slowly getting used to it. But now, you find yourself playing host to several other strange-sounding conditions, as well. Some of you may be affected by these conditions more than others; some not at all. Regardless, you'll need to learn more new terminology . . . again. If it makes you feel better, read only about those conditions affecting your life right now. You can always come back later to read about the other conditions if you need to. Keep in mind, the severity of these conditions can vary greatly from person to person—just as it can in scleroderma. If you feel you may actually have one of these conditions but have yet to be diagnosed, please check with your doctor before self-diagnosing. Many symptoms overlap among these conditions. Let your physician be the one to determine the cause of your symptoms.

As you read about these conditions, remember this: The following list includes only the most common accompanying conditions and doesn't include disease manifestations, or other, less common, conditions that you may experience. It is meant to educate you, not frighten you.

Hopefully, the following information will help to demystify those peculiar-sounding conditions so you're able to recognize and understand exactly what you're dealing with.

Raynaud's phenomenon

Occurring in approximately 90 to 95 percent of scleroderma patients, Raynaud's phenomenon is a disorder that affects the blood vessels in the fingers and toes, and much less commonly, the ears and nose. The underlying process is a decreased blood supply to the extremities, causing the blood vessels to spasm. Most commonly seen in the fingers, episodic attacks are characterized by skin color changes (white, blue, and red) and are usually triggered by exposure to cold or emotional stress. The order of the color changes varies from person to person and can produce throbbing, numbness, and/or a tingling sensation. An attack can last from less than a minute to up to several hours.

To take it a step further, Raynaud's phenomenon must be distinguished from primary Raynaud's disease. Primary Raynaud's disease is seen in approximately 5 to 10 percent of the adult population and is not associated with an underlying disease or other medical problems. But when Raynaud's is associated with another disease process, such as scleroderma, it's called secondary Raynaud's phenomenon.

TREATMENT OPTIONS

The treatment for Raynaud's phenomenon is aimed at trying to reduce both the number and severity of the attacks. This involves both medication and non-medication therapies.

Several of the non-medication treatments are the following:

1. *Keep yourself warm.* Make sure you are appropriately dressed in cold weather. Use gloves, mittens, extra socks, even hand warmers. And don't forget your hat. A good portion of your body heat is lost through your head. Be aware that air conditioning can also trigger an attack. Try to have a sweater handy if you're going to be in an air-conditioned place

for any length of time. And don't forget about the refrigerator either: Depending on the severity of your condition, it may be useful to put on gloves before handling frozen or refrigerated foods. Think ahead and think smart.

2. *Quit smoking.* Smoking only worsens the attacks, because the nicotine decreases blood flow to the fingers and toes. Just one more reason to quit that nasty habit.

3. *Try to control your stress.* Because emotional stress can trigger an attack, learn to recognize and avoid stressful situations as best you can. Many people have found that relaxation techniques or **biofeedback** training can help decrease both the number and severity of attacks.

4. *Keep your doctor informed.* If you find the attacks are increasing in frequency or resulting in sores or ulcers on your fingers or toes, you must let your doctor know. Only your doctor can determine the best treatment for you.

The medication treatments include

1. calcium channel blockers: This is the most commonly used treatment and believed to be the most effective.
2. nitroglycerin paste: This is applied directly to the fingers (or wherever needed) and helps open up the blood vessels.
3. vasodilators: This is used for patients who are unresponsive to calcium channel blockers.

Sjögren's syndrome

Sjögren's ("show-grins") syndrome occurs in approximately 20 to 25 percent of patients with scleroderma. Also classified as an autoimmune disease, Sjögren's targets the moisture-producing glands in the body. The end result is a feeling of dryness in the eyes, mouth, and vagina.

Some of the symptoms include

○ **dry eyes:** You may notice a dry, gritty feeling in your eyes or awaken to a dried, thick mucous in the corners of your eyes.

- ○ **dry mouth:** Because you are producing less saliva, speaking and eating may become more difficult. This symptom can also diminish your sense of taste.
- ○ **dry cough:** Another symptom you may notice is a persistent dry cough. This is called bronchitis **sicca.**
- ○ **dry vagina:** Vaginal dryness may result in vaginal irritation, as well as uncomfortable sexual intercourse.

The treatment for Sjögren's syndrome is aimed at alleviating the symptoms through artificial moisturizing methods to minimize their effects on your daily life. For example, dry eyes can be treated with artificial tears; dry mouth can be treated with over-the-counter saliva substitutes or gels. Sugar-free gum and candies help to stimulate saliva flow, and sips of water throughout the day help to alleviate the dry-mouth feeling. For vaginal dryness, you can use specially designed lubricants. Just make sure you don't use petroleum jelly or any oil-based products, as they will interfere with the vagina's natural cleansing process. If other areas are affected, please speak to your doctor to find out the best treatment for you.

I'd also like to point out that over 50 percent of scleroderma patients experience dry eyes and dry mouth unrelated to Sjögren's syndrome. As always, please check with your doctor to receive the proper diagnosis for your symptoms.

Sjögren's syndrome is rarely life-threatening and is easily managed with many of the over-the-counter moisturizing agents available.

Fibromyalgia

Fibromyalgia occurs in approximately 15 to 20 percent of scleroderma patients. According to Daniel J. Wallace and Janice Brock Wallace in their book *All About Fibromyalgia* (Oxford Press, 2002), fibromyalgia essentially is a form of chronic neuromuscular pain, or "pain-amplification syndrome." It is characterized by muscle pain, stiffness, and easy fatigability. Although the syndrome can occur spontaneously, in most cases it is associated with trauma or stress, or secondary to conditions such as scleroderma or lupus.

In order to be diagnosed with fibromyalgia, a patient must have

1. widespread pain of at least three months' duration;

2. pain in all four quadrants of the body: right side, left side, above the waist, and below the waist;
3. pain occurring in at least 11 of 18 specified "tender" points, with at least one point in each quadrant; and
4. pain defined as discomfort when 8 pounds of pressure are applied to the tender point.

Traditional treatments are aimed at improving quality of sleep as well as reducing pain. The most common medications used are NSAIDs (non-steroidal anti-inflammatory drugs) for pain, and tricyclic antidepressants or SSRIs, to help boost the body's level of **serotonin**. Other medications are available, too, and should be discussed with your rheumatologist.

Patients can also benefit from physical therapy, relaxation techniques, gentle exercise programs, and reduction of stress.

Overlap syndromes

Just because you have scleroderma doesn't mean you can't get another connective-tissue disease. In fact, it is estimated that as many as 20 to 30 percent of patients have an overlap syndrome. An **overlap syndrome** simply means having features of two or more diseases. While my own disease is predominantly scleroderma, I also test positive to **antibodies** found in lupus. The most common scleroderma overlap is with polymyositis, followed by rheumatoid arthritis and lupus. Just as it is in scleroderma, the treatment for overlap syndromes is aimed at controlling the underlying disease.

Overlap syndromes are not to be confused with undifferentiated connective-tissue disease. These patients don't classically fit the textbook diagnostic criteria of any one particular disease in the beginning but often go on later to develop a defined disease.

Other conditions

Other accompanying conditions can include **pulmonary hypertension** (10-15%), thyroid disease (20-30%), and primary biliary cirrhosis (5-10%). All come with their own sets of symptoms and treatments. If you're concerned about any of the above conditions, I urge you to speak to your rheumatologist as soon as possible. As you'll learn in Week 3, early intervention is crucial when treating both scleroderma and any other accompanying conditions.

Hopefully, you will not be affected by any of these conditions. But if you are, keep in mind that while some are merely nuisances, others can be life-threatening. Most of these conditions need to be managed with the same vigilance required in managing scleroderma. It may feel to you like a constant juggling act, but try to remember that your knowledge and understanding are key to successfully treating whatever additional conditions may come your way.

IN A SENTENCE:

Accompanying conditions are quite normal in scleroderma and often require additional treatments.

learning

Learning to Educate Yourself

GETTING SCLERODERMA is kind of like the first day of school. You walk in knowing absolutely nothing. But, with school, you have a teacher, whose sole purpose is to make sure you learn your ABCs. With scleroderma, unfortunately, there's no teacher to teach you the ABCs of scleroderma. That's up to you. Sure, you have your doctor. But the information you receive from your physician is usually transmitted on a "need to know" basis—hardly sufficient for those of us who desire more knowledge. Besides, your physician gets paid to treat your medical condition—not to teach you. So, where do you turn to educate yourself? I'll get to that a little later. More importantly, let's talk about *why* you need to.

Taking charge

As you learned in Day 3, people manage their disease in different ways. Some patients jump right in with both feet; others step back and take a "wait and watch" approach. We all need to approach things in a way that feels comfortable. But don't lose sight of what your ultimate goal is: to try to do everything in your power to help your doctor help you. Remember, this is a team effort. The more knowledgeable you become, the better able you are to make informed decisions on your own treatment and care. More importantly, gaining knowledge of scleroderma gives you a sense of control over your situation and empowers you to become your own advocate. Becoming your own advocate may be the single most important thing you can do for yourself as a patient. But this means taking a very active role in your medical care. For some of you, this role may come naturally, but for others, it may not come quite as easily. Here are a few suggestions on how you can become your own advocate.

1. ***Become an assertive patient.*** This doesn't mean becoming aggressive and pushy. This means

   ○ learning to feel comfortable asking your questions and expecting answers
   ○ asking for a further explanation if you don't understand the answer
   ○ knowing you deserve the best care instead of feeling surprised when you get it
   ○ learning to speak the doctor's language, so when you nod your head in agreement, you do so because you really do understand what your physician is saying
   ○ having the confidence to disagree with your physician and knowing that it's okay to do so
   ○ feeling free to speak your mind about how you feel about a situation, instead of saying what you think your physician wants to hear

2. ***Empower yourself through knowledge.*** This means not only learning about scleroderma, but learning about how scleroderma affects *you*. As you learned in Day 2, there are many different forms of the disease and every patient is affected differently. This is an overwhelming disease. The more you know about your particular manifestation of the disease, the more control you have in making informed decisions about your treatment.

3. ***Be a good listener.*** Part of being an educated patient is being a good listener. Try to use your time spent with your doctor as best you can, by paying attention and focusing on what's being said. You're paying your doctor for his or her advice; the least you can do is listen to it.

Becoming a "professional patient"

Now that you've learned why it's so important to educate yourself, let's talk about how to go about it. Early on in my diagnosis, I remember thinking how much time it took to be a patient with a chronic disease. Between the research, doctor appointments, and medical tests, I felt like I was in training to become a "professional patient"—only without the pay. Even though educating yourself may be time-consuming right now, I think you'll find it's time well spent, in the long run. Let's talk about the resources you can use, so that you too can train to become a "professional patient."

O   *Organizations*—The scleroderma world is made up of two foundations: the Scleroderma Foundation and the Scleroderma Research Foundation. Both are wonderful organizations and do an amazing job for the scleroderma community. In a perfect world, it would be advantageous to have the two foundations work together as one—but each organization has distinct and different goals. Let's take a look at what each foundation does and how they can help you.

1.   **The Scleroderma Foundation**—This is a national organization with 26 local chapters dedicated to people with scleroderma and their family and friends. It was formed in 1998 by a merger between West Coast–based United Scleroderma Foundation and the East Coast–based Scleroderma Federation. One of the first phone calls you make upon learning of your diagnosis should be to this foundation. The staff can provide you with educational pamphlets, patient support groups, physician referrals in your area, and much more. In addition, the foundation holds a national conference once a year, a Capitol Hill day in Washington, D.C., and educational symposia all over the country. The national office of the Scleroderma Foundation is in Byfield, Massachusetts, and can be reached at 800-722-HOPE (4673) or *www.scleroderma.org*. Its mission is threefold:

    O   *Support:* to help patients and their families cope with scleroderma through mutual support groups, peer counseling, physician referrals, and educational material

○ *Education:* to promote public awareness and education through health seminars, literature, and publicity campaigns

○ *Research:* to stimulate and support research in order to improve treatment and ultimately find the cause and cure of scleroderma and related diseases

2. **The Scleroderma Research Foundation (SRF)**—Established in 1987, and based in Santa Barbara, California, the SRF is the only organization focused exclusively on finding a cure for scleroderma. Through nationwide public awareness efforts and an innovative research approach, the SRF has raised millions of dollars for research over the years.

The organization has created two collaborative research centers whose focus is on high-quality, cutting-edge research. More specifically, the SRF is focused on research at the cellular level to understand the mechanisms of the disease and ultimately to develop therapies that stop or reverse its progress. If fundraising is your thing, this organization has a wonderful cure-advocate program that allows you to create your own fundraiser. Speaking from experience, I can attest that you actually *can* make a difference.

The Scleroderma Research Foundation can be reached at 800-441-CURE (2873) or *www.sclerodermaUSA.org.*

Although the Scleroderma Foundation focuses on patient support, education, and research, and the Scleroderma Research Foundation's focus is on research to find a cure, both organizations offer not only a wealth of information to learn from but also many opportunities to get involved. From cure-advocate programs to patient support groups, venues for getting involved not only provide you with a wonderful education, but also give you a sense of control over the many frustrations the disease can bring.

○ *Websites:* As you probably already know, you can find out about just about anything you want to on the Internet. A google search on scleroderma will lead you in a thousand different directions. The problem you'll confront is in evaluating a website's reliability. Use common sense and keep in mind that if something doesn't sound right to you, it probably isn't. You'll find the most reliable websites listed in the Resources section of this book. Here are a few other valuable Internet resources that you may not know about.

1. **MEDLINE**: This website is the U.S. National Library of Medicine's (NLM) premier database, containing over 12 million references to journal articles from over 4,600 worldwide journals. PubMed is the NLM's free search service, which allows access to MEDLINE through NLM's homepage at *www.nlm.nih.gov*. MEDLINE can also be reached through another very valuable resource: Medscape, a service from WebMD that features (in addition to MEDLINE) medical journal articles, case reports, medical news, major conference coverage, and comprehensive drug information. Medscape can be reached at *www.medscape.com*.

2. **Medication resource websites**: If you want to learn more about the medications you're taking, you may want to check out any of these websites: *www.rxlist.com*, *www.my.webmd.com*, and *www.drkoop.com*.

3. **Lab tests explained**: Want a better understanding of the lab tests you've just taken? Try *www.labtestsonline.org*. For a more detailed listing of the rheumatological lab tests, try *www.sclero.org/medical/general/tests/antibodies.html*.

4. **Scleroderma online messageboard**: The International Scleroderma Network (ISN) has a wonderful website that offers a messageboard and e-mail list. Go to ISN's homepage at *www.sclero.org* and then click on the Sclero MSN online support community link.

○ *Your pharmacist*: This is one resource patients often forget about. As you learned earlier, doctors may not know all the interactions of every drug you take. In fact, some doctors will even refer you to a pharmacist if they can't find what they're looking for in the *Physician Drug Reference* (PDR). I've become great friends with my pharmacist over the years. Not only has she helped me learn more about some of the new drugs that I have to take, and their interactions with each other;

she's also helped me to sort out some of the insurance snags that are part of everyday life in the pharmaceutical world.

○ *Books:* For the most comprehensive guide to scleroderma, written in lay terms from a physician's viewpoint, I highly recommend *The Scleroderma Book: A Guide for Patients and Families* by Maureen Mayes. She provides easy-to-understand explanations of all aspects of the disease, from the most mild form to the most severe.

○ *Other scleroderma patients:* One of the most frustrating aspects of this disease is actually finding someone who truly understands what you're going through. Other scleroderma patients not only offer you understanding and support, but can be a wonderful resource for new treatment options, physician recommendations, or symptom comparisons. If you don't have access to a computer to join an on-line forum, try your local support group. Reaching out and communicating with other patients will provide you with a hands-on education you won't find anywhere else.

Tricks of the trade

Congratulations: you're on your way to becoming a professional patient. Now that you've learned a few tricks of the trade, you'll find yourself becoming a more confident and educated patient. Just remember, learning is a lifelong process. Never forget to keep an open mind in your continued search for knowledge and answers.

IN A SENTENCE:

Educating yourself on all aspects of your disease is crucial in helping you to become your own advocate, and there are lots of resources available to help you along the way.

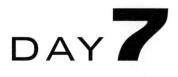
The Blues, the Blahs, and the Rest of Those Bad Feelings

HAVING A chronic illness means we are presented with a variety of new (a.k.a. bad) feelings, most of which we are ill-prepared to deal with. One day everything's fine, and the next we're being bombarded with a bevy of emotions we don't know what to do with. Shock, anger, horror, denial, self-pity, sadness, resentment, relief, fear, hopelessness, guilt . . . sound familiar? These feelings may come in stages or they may overwhelm you at once. But no matter the sequence or timing, let's get one thing straight: They're all normal feelings to be having right now. You've experienced a loss and are probably going through your own grieving process. You may have heard of Elisabeth Kübler-Ross's five stages of grief: denial, anger, bargaining, depression, and acceptance. Much has been written about these five stages, because it was thought that a healthy emotional outlook could only be achieved by going through each of these stages. But the reality is that no two people are going to react to the same news in the same way. And the intensity of one's feelings is really a reflection of how that loss or change is perceived. Not everyone is going to enter the grieving process in the same place or go through these stages in the same order. The bottom line? Allow yourself to feel whatever emotion you're feeling in whatever order it happens to come in. Your goal should be acceptance of your disease, the sooner you get there, the better. Now, that doesn't mean you should act as though these other feelings don't exist. On the contrary. I think it's vital to your emotional well-being that you allow yourself to feel these different feelings. And on some level, you may feel your loss for the rest of your life. That's okay, as long as you know what your goal is: acceptance of your disease. Now, let's figure out how to get there, even with all of these uncomfortable emotions.

Your emotions: the good, the bad, and the ugly

There have probably been, only a handful of times in your life when you've had to deal with so many different emotions at the same time. Some of your feelings may last longer than you think they should, and you may wonder if that's normal. Other emotions come and go so quickly you're not even sure you felt them. Let's talk about what some of those emotions are and how they can make you feel.

- ❍ **Fear** Fear is defined as anxiety caused by real or possible danger or pain. After your diagnosis, some things you may be fearful of include disease progression, change in appearance, losing your independence, loss of financial independence, pain, loss of control over your life, and of course, dying. Fear can be paralyzing. But if you take a closer look at what you're fearful of, you'll find you may have had some of these same fears even before you got your diagnosis. We all have a fear of dying, or a fear of pain. Only now, these fears are amplified by something very real and tangible. Although all your fears may be warranted right now, don't let them stop you from living your life today. We all live with fear every day. We need to address our fears and try to deal with them rationally. If we gave in to every fear we've ever had, we would never leave the house, let alone live a fulfilling life.
- ❍ **Anger** There's plenty of reason to be angry after being diagnosed with scleroderma. Your life as you know it is going to change

dramatically. And you find this horribly unfair. Your head begins to fill up with all sorts of questions, like "Why me?" or "What have I done wrong?" You begin to lash out at your loved ones for no reason and find yourself becoming incredibly short-tempered. Little things in your life that never used to bother you have become a huge source of frustration. Let's face it. Anger can be a nasty emotion. And it can be one of the most difficult to deal with. But the key to anger is to learn how to express it appropriately. Whether you turn to a therapist, a support group, a family member, or a good friend, find an outlet that allows you to safely express your anger. Some people find an outlet through exercise. Or perhaps by punching pillows. Whatever you do, try not to take it out on those closest to you. And don't try to suppress your anger either. Unexpressed anger can result in very real physical ailments, such as headaches and stomachaches. And you certainly don't need any additional physical problems on top of what you've got. It's okay to feel angry at your disease. Just try and figure out the best, most comfortable way to express it.

○ **Guilt** This is a very common emotion but one that doesn't necessarily belong here. You may feel as though an unhealthy lifestyle or a less-than-wholesome diet may have brought on your disease. Remember what you learned in Day 1? Getting scleroderma is not your fault. You didn't do anything wrong. Adding broccoli and berries to your diet wouldn't have made one bit of difference in where you are today. You may also feel a certain amount of guilt if you can't fulfill your responsibilities to your family or are feeling as though you're a burden to others. We've all felt that way at one time or another. But remember, you didn't ask to get a disease, so don't blame yourself because you did. Communicate your feelings with your family and let them know how you're feeling.

○ **Denial** This is a normal emotion and is most commonly felt right after diagnosis. It's essentially a defense mechanism we use to give ourselves more time to adjust to bad news. And, let's face it, who's ever ready to deal with the diagnosis of a chronic illness? Or to deal with the fact that we may not be able to work or do the things we used to do? It's a lot easier to pretend it's not happening. Denial is normal. But, although denial of your disease may help to relieve some of the anxiety you may be feeling right now, it can't last forever. Some of your disease manifestations may require immediate intervention. The longer you're in denial, the more your health may suffer. Take the time you need to accept your disease, but realize that sooner or later you won't be able to ignore your new reality. Your long-term health is at stake.

○ **Depression** Depression sometimes follows after the reality of your situation sets in. And it seems to be one of those emotions that can creep up on you out of nowhere. All of a sudden you find yourself crying all the time and feeling sorry for yourself. Nothing you do makes you happy anymore. And you're just generally feeling blah all the time. It can affect everything in your life, from eating and sleeping to just about anything else you do on a daily basis. Feelings of sadness are a normal reaction to the news of having a chronic illness. Hopefully, these feelings will subside after a short while. If you find you have prolonged feelings of hopelessness so severe you wonder if it's all worth it, then you need help. In addition to seeing a professional mental health counselor, you may need an antidepressant medication to help you. And if you feel you've reached the end of your rope, you need to contact your local suicide prevention hotline. Don't let your feelings of shame prevent you from getting the treatment you need. Depression can be treated. You just have to take the first step.

○ **Relief** Probably the only decent emotion of the bunch, relief comes after a lengthy diagnostic process (or even a short one). At last, the uncertainty is over. You finally have a name for all the strange symptoms you've been experiencing and are relieved to know you're not crazy after all. Temporarily, you're thrilled—not because you were diagnosed with a chronic disease, but because now you know you will get the treatment you need to begin to feel better. And that's a huge relief.

○ **Shame** Some may view their illness as a weakness and feel ashamed to have a disease. You're used to being strong, independent, and in control. Now you feel inadequate. And weak. It's true, your body may be weaker than it was before you got scleroderma. But your mind isn't. Having a disease is nothing to be ashamed of. Don't get trapped in the mindset that you are any less of a person just because you got sick.

How to cope with these bad feelings

When confronted with these types of feelings, there's definitely a healthy and an unhealthy way to cope. One patient I spoke with went into a deep depression for over ten years after her diagnosis. Her depression, she says, was caused by the changes she had to make in her lifestyle due to the disease. She turned to drugs and alcohol to help her cope with her depression, which only made her feel worse. She's doing better these days, with the help of medication, but continues to battle her depression on a daily basis.

All of these different emotions can wreak havoc on your self-esteem, not to mention your daily life. Sometimes all you need to know is that you're not alone with these feelings and that other patients have felt the same way. In this situation, a support group may be the best thing for you. You can read more about support groups in the Learning section of Week 4. But if you find any of the above emotions are interfering with the way you live your life, you may need medical intervention to help you cope. Speak to your physician about taking antianxiety or antidepressant medication. If you decide to take an antidepressant, you may have to try several types before finding the one that works for you. This is normal. Once you've discovered the right one for you, give the medication a chance to work and it can make a world of difference in how you feel. In conjunction with the medication, some people may benefit from talking about their feelings with a mental health professional. Others may feel more comfortable in talking to a counselor *without* taking any medication. There is no right or wrong solution. The best solution is one that works for you and your lifestyle.

You may need to experience all of these emotions before you get to your ultimate goal of acceptance. Or you may only experience one. Just know what your goal is and that there is plenty of help out there to help you achieve it. It may take some time, but you will get there.

IN A SENTENCE:

> *It's normal to go through many different emotions before you can ultimately accept your disease.*

learning

Your Emotional Journey

GETTING A diagnosis of a chronic illness wreaks havoc on just about every aspect of your life. Because most of your focus in these early days is on the physical aspects of your new disease, emotional aspects may get pushed aside. It seems most people are more interested in finding a cure for their disease than in learning to live with their feelings and their illness. It isn't until much later in the process that you stop and think about how your disease is emotionally affecting you. You learned, in the Living section of this chapter, about the most common emotions you may experience; this section focuses on learning to live with those emotions on a daily basis.

In the early days of your diagnosis

At this point, you may still be feeling numb from your diagnosis. Maybe the news hasn't sunk in yet, and you're still running on adrenaline. But eventually, those feelings will come about, tap you on the shoulder, and make you address them straight on. As unpleasant and uncomfortable as it sounds, this is actually a good thing. The sooner you begin to deal with the swirl of emotions you're feeling, the sooner you can begin to accept your new life with a chronic illness. Many people will go out of their way to avoid feeling negative emotions. They continually deny the truth to themselves, which can result in their engaging in bizarre and destructive behavior. Don't let your emotions get the best of you. Negative and anxious emotions, if suppressed, torment not only the mind, but the body—not to mention your spirit. And don't forget the long-term effects negative emotions can have. You'll read more about how this type of stress can affect your body and disease in Month 10.

Try not to have unrealistic expectations of yourself

Just as no two people are affected physically by scleroderma in the same way, so they react differently, emotionally. Some people may cry for weeks on end upon getting their diagnosis; others may never shed a tear. But, it doesn't necessarily mean these two people aren't feeling the same emotion. They probably are. They're just expressing it differently. While it may be of some comfort to hear how other patients are coping with their emotions, it's more important not to compare yourself emotionally with others. You need to experience your own feelings in your own way and your own time frame. Don't get caught up in the amount of time it may take you to get through a particular feeling or "stage." Don't be too hard on yourself when you're feeling down. Just know that if the negative feeling lasts longer than you're comfortable with, it may be wise to seek help. Same goes for any behavior or excessive lifestyle changes you may experience. Let yourself feel what you need to feel, but understand yourself well enough to know when to get help.

About your journey

All journeys begin with a single step. And your emotional journey is no different. Your emotional journey probably began before you even got your diagnosis. The frustration, the fear, the anxiety of not knowing what was wrong—all these emotions were just the beginning of a journey you didn't know you were about to take. But now your journey's begun. And you must learn to take it day by day, because every day is different. Maybe you got some bad news today about a test you took last week or maybe a troublesome new symptom popped up. But then the next day, your new symptom seems to have disappeared, or you realize your test results were not so bad after all. All this up and down can make you feel like you're on an emotional rollercoaster. You're not alone. All scleroderma patients go through these daily ups and downs. The difference lies in how much these ups and downs seem to affect your life. And your emotional journey becomes just that: your reaction to the impact of scleroderma on your daily life.

Take charge of your emotions

The emotional aspects of your disease can be just as important as the physical aspects. It's best not to let your emotions get the best of you, but there are times when you just can't help it. Sometimes you scream or become angrier than you'd like. Or you become irritable and impatient and begin to take out your anger on those around you who least deserve it. We've all done these things—they are common reactions to feeling overwhelmed by your emotions. But there are better ways to express your emotions. Let's take a look at some different ways of channeling your emotions more positively.

- ○ **Exercise**—Whether it's walking, swimming, tai chi, or yoga, find an activity that feels comfortable to you. It doesn't have to be strenuous. If you're not up to exercising, find a sturdy pillow to pound. You'd be surprised at how much better you feel after physically letting loose some of those angry emotions. Those closest to you will be grateful as well.
- ○ **Writing**—Those who keep daily journals swear by them. A journal doesn't have to be anything fancy; any pad of paper will do. Keeping a daily journal allows you to unburden negative feelings in the most private of ways. You can write down your innermost feelings and nobody but you will ever know what they are. If you can no longer write, try using a tape recorder. The point is to be able to express your private thoughts and get them off your chest. Feel uncomfortable about keeping a written journal around? Remember, you can always throw it away afterward.
- ○ **Art**—I recently read a magazine article about a man who was diagnosed with a terminal illness. His best friend felt helpless when he heard the news of the diagnosis and thought the best way to help his friend was to help him learn to express his emotions. The friend

bought two huge canvases and plenty of paint, and brought them to his sick friend. The two immediately sat down and began painting together. The terminally ill man had tears in his eyes when he thanked his friend for one of the most thoughtful gifts he had ever received. Most of us don't immediately think of art when we want to express our emotions. We're so used to expressing ourselves through talking, we seldom think to use a more creative process to express painful, negative emotions. The best thing about art is that you don't have to be the slightest bit "artistic" to gain the emotional benefits it can provide. What's important in artistic expression is the process, not the end result. Art can be a very powerful healing tool, whether you create an image through drawing, painting, sculpture, or collage. Just figure out what type of art you enjoy, make a trip to the art-supply store, and you're on your way to a new means of emotional expression and release.

- ○ **Hobbies**—When you feel like you're at the end of your rope, try to shift gears. Do something you enjoy doing. Sometimes the mere fact of shifting your focus allows you to feel calmer and to see things more clearly. And doing something you enjoy allows you to get a different perspective on what's going on in your life. Besides, we could all use a little more enjoyment in our lives.

- ○ **Talking**—While there are many forms of emotional expression, talking is the most common, and often the most comfortable. But you must choose a listener whom you trust and who is nonjudgmental. A good listener will do just that: listen. That may be all you need right now. The impact of scleroderma on your emotional stability is enormous. Although you may feel embarrassed at the depth of your emotion as you begin talking about scleroderma, don't be. Talking about these emotions can be incredibly therapeutic. Just make sure you talk about them regularly, to avoid keeping them bottled up inside you.

Take responsibility for your emotional health

Your emotional health needs the same amount of attention as your physical health. And it's up to you to provide it. Just being aware of the fact that your journey is an emotional one as well as a physical one is good place to start. Your emotions will need plenty of nurturing during your medical odyssey. Be sure you're paying attention to your needs so that you can take good care of them.

IN A SENTENCE:

Your emotional journey is just as important as your physical journey.

FIRST-WEEK MILESTONE

By the end of your first week, you have begun to take control of your scleroderma, as you have now

○ LEARNED EXACTLY WHAT SCLERODERMA IS AND ITS MANY DIFFERENT TYPES;

○ FIGURED OUT THE BEST WAY TO MANAGE YOUR DISEASE, IN A STYLE THAT'S RIGHT FOR YOU;

○ DISCOVERED HOW TO COPE WITH THE MANY PHYSICAL CHANGES THE DISEASE MAY BRING;

○ RECOGNIZED THE IMPORTANCE OF YOUR RHEUMATOLOGIST AND HOW TO ASSEMBLE YOUR MEDICAL TEAM;

○ BEEN EDUCATED ABOUT THE VARIOUS CONDITIONS THAT CAN ACCOMPANY SCLERODERMA AND THE IMPORTANCE OF EDUCATING YOURSELF; AND

○ REALIZED THAT YOUR FEELINGS OF SHOCK, FEAR, AND ANGER ARE NORMAL AND THAT YOU ARE NOT ALONE.

Tests, Tests, and More Tests—What You Need and Why

IT'S BEEN a long couple of weeks. You finally have a diagnosis and are dealing with the reality of living with a chronic disease. You're tired of seeing doctor after doctor and want to take
a little breather. Hold that thought. You're going to need to wait
a little longer. Just because you've received your diagnosis doesn't
mean the testing stops. In fact, for some people, it's just the
beginning. When your symptoms first began, your physician
may have run some routine blood work. He or she probably ran
a complete blood count (CBC), which analyzes red cells, white
cells, and platelets. It's one of the most commonly performed
blood tests in the United States. But that's just the starting
point. Scleroderma is a very complicated disease, necessitating
more than just routine lab work. You may also need specialized
tests to determine any internal organ involvement. It would be
nearly impossible to give you a list of tests that apply to every
scleroderma patient. Your particular symptoms will determine
which tests you need. You'll learn more about organ-specific testing later in this chapter. For now, let's talk about the process.

In the beginning

Let's say you've been given a diagnosis of sclerodema, based on your clinical evaluation as well as some abnormal laboratory results. More specifically, your **antinuclear antibody (ANA)** test, a basic screening test for autoimmune diseases, is abnormal. You're then sent to a rheumatologist for further evaluation. At this point, several things need to be evaluated.

1. A more definitive diagnosis needs to be made, to confirm your scleroderma diagnosis and to rule out any overlap syndromes.
2. The extent of internal organ damage needs to be assessed.
3. More extensive antibody panels need to be taken.

Let's start with the blood work. Most doctors will order the following lab work upon diagnosis:

○ *Complete blood count*—Yep, even though you just had one done, most doctors like to have another done at the lab of their choice. Some doctors won't trust tests taken by another doctor and/or lab. This doesn't make much sense, but get used to it. The propensity can become a particular (not to mention costly) nuisance if you change doctors a lot. Each time you see a new one, you'll most likely have to repeat some, if not all, blood work.

○ *Blood chemistry panel*—Often called a comprehensive metabolic profile, this panel evaluates many things, such as kidney function, liver function, blood sugar, and electrolytes. The lipid profile looks at your total cholesterol, including triglycerides, HDL, and LDL; the thyroid panel looks at your thyroid function by testing T3, T4, and TSH. Inflammatory indices such as CPK, Sed Rate, and CRP are also ordered and evaluated. There can also be additional studies ordered, such as iron levels or pancreatic function tests. The specific types of tests you'll need will be determined by your physician.

○ *Antibody screening*—Once it's determined that your ANA is positive, another set of antibody panels is ordered. Once again, exactly which tests are ordered will be determined by your physician. The specific scleroderma antibody tests include

1. **antinuclear antibody (ANA)**—This test is positive in about 95 percent of patients. Further testing may be done to evaluate the pattern.
2. **antitopoisomerase antibody (Anti-Scl-70)**—This test is positive in about 25 percent of patients with diffuse disease and in 5 to 10 percent of patients with limited disease.
3. **anticentromere antibody**—This test is positive in approximately 10 to 15 percent with diffuse disease and about 60 to 90 percent with limited disease.

○ *Additional panels*—If your doctor suspects you may have an overlap syndrome, the following antibody tests will be ordered: **Antibody to ribonucleoprotein (Anti-RNP), Ro antibody (Anti-SSA),** and rheumatoid factor. In addition, if you're experiencing any out-of-the-ordinary symptoms (for scleroderma, that is), your doctor will probably order more extensive antibody testing. Unfortunately, these tests tend to be more expensive, take longer to perform, and should only be sent to very experienced immunologic laboratories.

In addition to the above lab tests, you'll also have the following tests:

○ *Urinalysis*—This test screens for any urinary tract infections or kidney disease. It can also screen for diseases of other organs that result in abnormal metabolites appearing in the urine. Specifically, the urine is tested for protein, glucose, hemoglobin, ketones, acidity, and specific gravity.
○ *Blood pressure*—A baseline must be taken and then checked periodically, as a rapid increase in blood pressure can indicate kidney disease.

A few other tests may be ordered just to get baseline results. These include a chest X-ray and an echocardiogram. If any lung involvement is suspected, your physician may also order some lung function tests; you'll read more about those specific tests in the lung section of this chapter.

These tests are all routine, so don't freak out

I know, I know . . . you're already sick of all the testing and are feeling like an oversized pincushion. It's all so time-consuming and you're not convinced it's all really necessary. Is it? Yes. As much as you may dislike being poked and prodded, your doctor is only doing his or her job, and what's best for you. This is the time your doctor must be thorough, and that necessitates a complete evaluation of your condition. The results of these tests will help your doctor determine how severe your disease is, and the best course of action to take. And, unfortunately, that can often mean more testing. If your doctor is concerned about any organ involvement (kidneys, lungs, GI tract), you'll most likely need to see a specialist, who will probably order more testing to be done. This is where it can get particularly frustrating. Not only is your rheumatologist involved in your tests, but now you have other specialists involved, all ordering their own tests and interpreting the results.

To help keep your focus, here's a tip: Remember what you learned in Day 5? Your rheumatologist is your quarterback. It's crucial that all your doctors are sharing your test results with the person in charge. And that's your rheumatologist. If they're not, it's up to you to make sure it happens. Your other doctors are organ specialists, not disease specialists. Your rheumatologist must be involved in all decisions about your treatment. That said, let's look at what other tests you may need if your physician suspects you have organ involvement.

Lung tests

- ○ *Chest X-ray*—Easy and inexpensive, this test is usually performed routinely upon diagnosis.
- ○ *CT (CAT) scan*—If the X-ray appears normal but lung involvement is suspected, a special high-resolution CAT scan is performed to further evaluate your lungs.
- ○ *Pulmonary function tests (PFTs)*—These tests assess lung breathing capacities, evaluate **interstitial** lung function, and measure the efficiency of gas exchange across the pulmonary membrane.
- ○ *Bronchoscopy*—If a biopsy of your lung tissue is needed, this procedure is performed through a flexible, thin tube passed into your lungs.

○ **Bronchoalveolar lavage (BAL)**—Also done during the bronchoscopy, this procedure is a washing of the cells taken from your lungs to analyze the cell types present in your lung tissue.

○ **Pulse oximetry**—A noninvasive test that measures how well the body is saturating oxygen while breathing.

○ **Arterial blood gases (ABGs)**—Blood is taken from an artery instead of a vein to measure how much oxygen is flowing through the arteries.

○ **Lung scans**—Nuclear medicine studies used for a variety of diagnostic purposes—one of which is to rule out a pulmonary embolus (blood clot).

○ **Two-dimensional (2D) doppler echocardiogram—Ultrasound** of the heart to measure and estimate pulmonary pressures.

○ **Pulmonary angiogram**—The "gold standard" procedure used for diagnosing pulmonary hypertension, it is also used to diagnose a pulmonary embolus.

Kidney tests

○ **Blood tests**—Creatinine and blood urea nitrogen (BUN) are the most common lab tests to evaluate kidney function.

○ **Urinalysis**—This will check for blood and protein as well as any other casts in the urine.

○ **24-hour urine protein**—If protein is found in the urine, this test will be ordered to quantitate the amount. Creatinine clearance will also be evaluated.

○ **Kidney ultrasound**—Used to evaluate the size and shape of kidneys.

○ **Blood pressure**—Easy test used to monitor blood pressure on a regular basis, to help to avoid malignant phase hypertension.

○ **Kidney biopsy**—Used to confirm diagnosis, evaluate kidney tissue, and determine treatment.

Heart tests

○ **Echocardiogram**—Ultrasound of the heart used to measure heart function. It examines how well the chambers are pumping and how well the heart valves are working. This test is also used to look for pericardial effusions (fluid around the sac of the heart), commonly seen in scleroderma.

○ *Electrocardiogram (EKG or ECG)*—A noninvasive test used to measure heart rate, rhythm, and chamber size.

○ *Holter monitor*—A portable EKG monitor worn for 24 hours to check for heart rhythm abnormalities.

○ *Cardiac stress test*—Usually performed on a treadmill, this test determines if the heart is getting adequate blood during exercise.

○ *Cardiac catheterization*—A procedure used to measure pressures in the heart and the pulmonary artery. Also used to determine if any vessels are blocked.

GI tract tests

○ *Endoscopy*—A procedure used to evaluate the lining of the esophagus and stomach.

○ *Barium swallow*—An upper GI X-ray procedure used to evaluate the esophagus.

○ *Hydrogen breath study*—A test done to determine if there is bacteria in the small bowel and to check for **malabsorption**.

○ *Upper GI series*—A barium swallow that can help to evaluate problems in the stomach and the small bowel.

○ *Esophagram*—An X-ray test taken to evaluate the motion of the esophagus.

○ *Transit study*—A nuclear medicine study used to measure the time it takes for the food to go from the stomach through to the bowel. Also called a gastric emptying study.

○ *Colonoscopy*—An invasive procedure used to evaluate the large bowel.

As I've mentioned elsewhere, just because a test is listed here does not mean you need it. The above is merely a list of some of the most common diagnostic tests that may be ordered for a particular organ. However, if your medical team does decide you need further testing, this is the time to be your own best advocate. Make sure you ask the following questions of the physician: Why are you ordering this test? Do you suspect a problem or just want a baseline result? What can I expect from the actual test? When will I get the results?

If you feel your situation warrants a further explanation, make sure you ask any other questions you may need answers to. Going through a lot of testing can cause tremendous anxiety. Make sure you feel comfortable with the process, to help alleviate any unnecessary stress.

IN A SENTENCE:

> *Your condition may necessitate many different types of tests, especially in the beginning.*

learning

The Importance of Early Treatment and Intervention

THERE'S NO doubt about it, scleroderma can be a very time-consuming disease. Especially in the beginning. As you learned in the Living part of this chapter, the amount of testing can become quite extensive and complicated, and can cause great anxiety. Not knowing what to expect from the tests, waiting for test results, and fear of the unknown lead to a very stressful situation. But the anxiety over *not* knowing what's going on can often be worse than the anxiety caused by the results. Wouldn't you rather know the facts? All this testing serves a much bigger purpose than creating inconvenience. Although you may not like all the results you get, at least you'll know the facts. And having all the facts allows you to actively seek the help you need.

Is it all really necessary?

Testing is not only time-consuming but also quite costly. You're probably asking yourself, "Why must I go through this?

Does it have to be done right now?" For one thing, you should remind your-self that you were just diagnosed with a chronic, often progressive, incurable disease. If that doesn't make you realize the necessity and importance of the testing, think about this: Without some of these tests, you may lose the function of one of your organs. That's right. Especially if you went through a lengthy diagnostic process. A lengthy diagnostic process means you're even that much further into the disease process. If your physician suspects any type of organ involvement, it's imperative to follow through with the testing ordered to determine the extent of the damage. Only then can you begin to treat the organ and hopefully prevent further damage.

Enough, already

You're still dragging your feet but are starting to realize how important this process is. You're exhausted from the disease and now you're exhausted by the procedures. The good news? Certain tests that are performed right now are simply to get a baseline assessment. That means once you're done with the test, it may not have to be repeated for a long time. Other tests, however, will require follow-up. For example, say your physician orders a chest X-ray and the results reveal something questionable. You can pretty much count on the fact that you'll need more tests. Your physician will probably order another test to confirm the results from the X-ray. If the diagnostic picture is still unclear, he or she will order another. This is the best way to uncover the facts. In a disease like scleroderma, the earlier you know the facts, the better.

Organ involvement in systemic disease

The statistics vary greatly as to who will and will not develop organ involvement. And the onset of internal organ development is highly unpredictable. For example, some doctors tell their patients that if they were to develop kidney disease, it would happen within the first five years of diagnosis. Then along comes a patient ten years into her or his diagnosis with classic signs of kidney damage. Doctors can't play God. Prognosis is based upon hundreds or thousands of other patients who have had the disease. This statistical information provides physicians with a general idea of what to expect. With a disease like scleroderma, however, it is important to note that no two patients are alike. Statistics from very large groups of people don't always accurately predict what will happen to a particular patient. Some physicians say that lung and GI involvement tends to occur within the first few years; but then again, it can happen anytime. What's a patient to do? The most any patient can do is to be monitored closely by their physician for the development or worsening of any internal organ involvement. That monitoring starts right now. If you were just diagnosed with systemic disease, make sure your doctor has taken some baseline tests to rule out asymptomatic organ involvement. The earlier you know what's going on, the better your chances for preventing permanent tissue or organ damage. Keep in mind that when your clinical picture is not clear-cut, more tests will be ordered to help sort things out. When I was going through this process, I complained bitterly to my friends and family about having to go through so many tests, day in and day out. It wasn't until much later in the process that I realized these tests might be saving my life.

But, my doctor didn't order any tests

You know in your gut that something isn't right. You've been complaining about some odd gastrointestinal problems for quite some time but never connected it to scleroderma. You tell your physician about it, but he or she blows it off, blaming it on the stress of the diagnosis, or perhaps your overindulgence in junk food. The doctor almost convinces you that there's nothing to worry about, so you cut back on your chocolate and caffeine intake—but then you're still not feeling better. Here's your chance to be a proactive patient. You know your body best. Listen to your instincts. If something doesn't feel right, it probably isn't. You need to have a frank discussion with your physician and ask either for some tests to be taken or for a referral to a gastroenterologist. And, even after you've been sent to a specialist, you may need to be more assertive than you'd like. I know, because it happened to me. After my diagnosis, I was experiencing severe GI problems and was sent to a gastroenterologist. He knew about my scleroderma diagnosis and after listening to my symptoms, he ordered exactly one test. Afterward, he diagnosed me as having irritable bowel disease. Although he claimed to know all about the complications of scleroderma, he refused to consider beyond the easiest and quickest "garbage can" diagnosis, as they say. In my gut (no pun intended), I knew immediately this was not the right diagnosis.

But when I brought this up, I was told that further testing would be a waste of time. Well, that was the end of that doctor. But I didn't stop there. I returned to my rheumatologist and was sent to another specialist. This time I was sent to a gastroenterologist who specialized in **motility** disorders, a common scleroderma GI complication. After two straight weeks of testing, this doctor was able to diagnose five separate GI complications attributable to scleroderma and started me on a medication regime that I take to this day. I felt very thankful that I had found him and that I had had the good sense to seek further attention for my symptoms. Being assertive can really pay off. If you know in your heart that your doctor isn't being as thorough as you'd like, keep pushing. You have nothing to lose and everything to gain.

Sometimes, disease progression to vital organs is inevitable, even with early intervention. But if you have the chance to be proactive about your disease, do it. Not only will you get a sense of control over your disease, but you'll have the peace of mind of knowing that you've done everything you possibly can to help yourself. The earlier you know about the complications from the disease, the greater your chances are for a better outcome.

The benefits of early intervention

Early diagnosis and treatment can decrease the chance of permanent tissue or organ damage. Period. Early intervention can even reduce the amount of time you spend on high-dose medication. But, as you've seen above, it may take some assertiveness on your part to get the ball rolling. Some doctors may stop just a test short of uncovering the real problem. Or you may feel not that you're getting too few tests, but that you're being put through unnecessary, costly, and time-consuming testing. The reality is you have a chronic, often progressive disease. Your goal is to work closely with your physician and medical team to uncover any hidden agendas your disease may have for you. And the earlier the better. That's not to say that just because something doesn't show up now, it won't pop up down the road. But all research indicates that early intervention can prevent further complications later. Taking an active role in your health care is a necessity in scleroderma. You're the boss. You know when a new symptom pops up or when that new medication isn't doing the trick anymore. Don't be afraid to speak up. And if you don't understand why your doctor did or didn't order that new test, make sure you ask why. You have a right to know. The more informed you are as a patient, the better able you are to monitor your own disease.

IN A SENTENCE:

> *Early treatment and intervention is essential in scleroderma to prevent further complications down the road.*

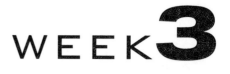
Why So Many Meds?

HAVE YOU ever seen those weekly pill organizers in drug-stores that hold up to a week's worth of pills and wonder who in the world uses those? Wonder no more. It only takes having to ingest more than a few pills a day to recognize the necessity of those little holders. I, personally, couldn't survive without mine. And sometimes I even think about getting the single AM/PM holder as well—anything to help keep my medications organized. At first, the whole pill-taking thing was incredibly overwhelming. I felt like I was 90 years old. "Take with meals"; "take after eating"; "take on an empty stomach"; "take before bedtime"; "take 4 times a day" . . . there seemed to be so many instructions that I wouldn't have blinked an eye if the label had said "take every two hours while standing on your head or take only when the moon is full." You begin to feel like a professional pill popper (a.k.a. addict). Somehow, you do get used to it, though, and it becomes just another part of your day. Even my family got used to it. My kids knew from the time they were very little not to touch Mommy's pills. As my kids got older, I thought it best not to have my pills seem so mysterious to them. The pills became such a normal part of our lives that, at the beginning of each week, as I organized my pills into their daily holders, my daughter was right there helping me get organized.

She loved to separate them by color and shape. But it wasn't always this way. I used to not like to take my pills in front of my kids. I used to think, "God, they'll think I'm sick *all* the time." Then one day, my kids asked the question. "Mom, why do you have to take so many pills every day?" I was caught off guard—and the answer I gave them surprised even me. I said, "Because they keep me well." That answer helped all of us see the positive side of taking all those pills.

Your new reality

As you've learned by now, there is no cure for scleroderma. But you can treat its symptoms. And that can mean taking many different pills to treat many different problems. Welcome to your new reality. Maybe you need to take a daily aspirin. Or an anti-inflammatory once a week. Or, perhaps you need heartburn medication twice a day, or an ACE inhibitor to help your kidneys. Keep in mind that whatever class of drug you need, your doctor has prescribed it for a reason. Whether to make you feel better now or to prevent further complications, taking pills will undoubtedly become part of your daily life if you have the systemic form of the disease. You'll learn more about the different types of treatment in the Learning section of this chapter.

Why you need them

Medications can be taken for all sorts of reasons: to treat the symptoms of the disease, to get rid of an infection, to combat the side effects of other drugs, or simply to slow the progression of the disease. One of the most frustrating situations you may encounter is when you need to take extra pills to combat the side effects of another medication. This has happened to me on several occasions. At one point in my disease, I had to go through six monthly infusions of a drug called Cytoxan to treat my lungs. Cytoxan is an **immuno-suppressive** therapy (a doctor's more "delicate" term for chemotherapy) used to treat many different types of cancer. Because of the side effects caused by this one medication, I found myself needing to take at least three other medications. All in all, it added an additional eight medications to my daily pill-popping routine. All this just to combat the side effects of one drug. Now, taking this many additional pills isn't typical for all medications. But if you find yourself having to take any immunosuppressive medications, you'll need to work closely with your physician to combat the side effects associated with that particular medication. Sometimes, it seems like a vicious cycle. The chemotherapy I'm on now causes both high blood pressure and high cholesterol. It seems the snowball effect never ends: Once again, I'm being closely monitored to make sure I won't need additional medications to combat these new side effects.

The Psychological Impact of "Popping Pills"

I USED to be the type of person who didn't even like to take an aspirin. Then I became a scleroderma patient, and I was popping pills like they were candy. At various points throughout my disease, I would get so sick of the pill-popping regime that I would just stop taking the pills. Boy, talk about big mistakes. Not only did I feel a lot crummier without the medications, but I learned from my doctor just how dangerous it can be to suddenly stop certain medications instead of slowly weaning off them. Don't ever stop your medications without speaking to your doctor first. I learned that lesson the hard way. But I did learn something positive. Part of the reason I wanted to stop taking the pills was that I believed I had to take the pills because I was sick. It wasn't until my kids asked me why I had to take so many pills that I realized the real reason I was taking them: to keep me well. Psychologically, that distinction can make a big difference in how you view your situation.

The importance of being a compliant patient

Your pills won't do you a bit of good if they stay in their bottles. Your doctor has prescribed these pills for a reason. The least you can do is to try to be a compliant patient. That means taking the pills in the way they were prescribed for whatever length of time they were prescribed for. Know why you're taking them and what they're for. And when you pick up your pills from the pharmacist, be a cautious consumer. Medication errors happen all the time. You, the patient, are the final link in the process. Being alert and knowledgeable allows you to be the last line of defense in preventing medication errors. Make sure you were given the right medication and the right dosage. And make sure you're aware of adverse effects, as well as drug and food interactions. You can play a vital role in preventing errors by asking questions and seeking satisfactory answers about your medication before it's dispensed.

Ever hear your doctor speak to a pharmacist about how to dose a medication? Here's the lowdown on dosing language, in lay terms:

QD = once a day
BID = twice a day
TID = three times a day
QID = four times a day

Once you begin your medication, it's up to you to report any unusual side effects or drug interactions you may be having. Reactions to medication vary from person to person. While it's up to the doctor to devise your treatment strategy, it's up to you to follow through.

Get to know your pharmacist

As you learned in Day 6, part of learning to educate yourself is learning about your medication. One resource vital to this process is your pharmacist. Not only can your pharmacist provide you with more in-depth information about your medication, but he or she can fill in the blanks that your doctor left empty.

Say your doctor prescribes a new medication and when you pick it up, you realize the pills are too big for you to swallow. This is the time to talk to your pharmacist. Your pharmacist will be able to tell you whether the medication is available in a smaller size or if it comes in an oral suspension (liquid) formula. You may even be able to cut the pills in half. But never cut your medication before checking with your pharmacist. Some pills come in capsule form or are time-released and should not be tampered with. If your pharmacist is unable to come up with a solution, you might want to talk to your doctor about using a compounding pharmacy. A compounding pharmacy is a specialized pharmacy that prepares customized medication for patients. Manufactured medications are wonderful but they don't always meet the individual needs of every patient. Some of the services a compounding pharmacy may provide include

1. customized medication strength;
2. preparation of special formulations to provide alternative delivery routes (some examples include **transdermal** creams, lozenges, capsules, suppositories, and lollipops);
3. custom flavoring of medications;
4. creation of formulas free of preservatives, fillers, and dyes, which may cause allergic reactions;
5. preparation of medications that are no longer available; and/or
6. combining ingredients into one dosage form, to simplify your medication schedule.

To find a reputable compounding pharmacy in your area, call the Professional Compounding Centers of America (PCCA). The PCCA is the largest association of compounding pharmacies in North America and can be reached at 800-331-2498 or at *www.ppcarx.com*.

Sometimes I feel as though I see my pharmacist more than my own family. We've actually become quite good friends. She's offered a wealth of information about possible drug interactions. And she's a whiz at working out insurance complications. Sometimes it really pays to get to know your pharmacist. You can rest assured you'll get better service at each visit. And when you visit your pharmacy as much as I do, that can make a big difference in your life.

IN A SENTENCE:

> *Taking many different types of medication is very common in a disease like scleroderma.*

learning

Treatment Options

WE ALL know by now there is no cure for scleroderma, but the good news is that there are many medications available to treat its symptoms. Because of the many different forms of the disease, it would be nearly impossible (not to mention irresponsible) for me to adeqately describe what treatment might be best for you. To determine what treatment you may need, you must work closely with your physician to devise a treatment strategy that's best for your particular disease manifestations. That's not to say we can't talk about treatment in a broader sense. A good place to start would be to talk about the three biological processes of scleroderma:

1. Vascular disease
2. **Autoimmunity**
3. Tissue fibrosis

Although most research is directed toward these three pathways, some doctors would argue there's a fourth disease process as well: inflammation. But regardless of the process, the goal remains the same: Overall treatment strategies should be aimed at targeting any or all of these disease processes. Once your doctor has determined the type of scleroderma you have, he or she can determine the activity of the disease process and any internal organ involvement you may have. Only after this evaluation is completed can your doctor recommend a specific treatment strategy for your particular disease.

The reality of disease-modifying drugs

You're probably asking yourself, Just what exactly is a disease-modifying drug? Essentially, it's a medication that would prevent or improve internal organ involvement, slow or reverse skin thickening, improve survival, lessen disability, and improve overall quality of life. Sounds too good to be true, right? Unfortunately, it is. At present, there are no medications that have been approved by the FDA or that have demonstrated any significant clinical evidence to modify the course of scleroderma. But that's not to say we don't use disease-modifying drugs to treat the disease. According to Daniel Furst, Carl M. Pearson Professor of Rheumatology at UCLA, the most commonly used drugs currently available to modify the course of scleroderma are methotrexate, D-penicillamine, cyclophosphamide, and steroids. Although all these medications have distinct purposes, the truth is that each one is as controversial as the next in treating the disease. Not only do these medications have serious side effects, but few have been properly evaluated for efficacy. That said, let's take a closer look at the reality of each of these drugs.

METHOTREXATE

This is an immunosuppressive drug often used to treat rheumatoid arthritis. Used to reduce inflammation, its use in scleroderma has had varied results, at best. But, of all the medications mentioned above, methotrexate at least has some scientific evidence behind it. According to Philip Clements, clinical professor of medicine at UCLA, "Methotrexate is the only medication that has controlled evidence that it may actually do anything for early diffuse disease—even though the trials were very small."

D-PENICILLAMINE

Used to weaken collagen, this drug used to be quite popular in treating scleroderma. Unfortunately, though, it hasn't proven to be quite the wonder drug everyone originally thought it was. Although a minority of scleroderma experts still use it, its efficacy has not been supported by a randomized, controlled trial.

CYCLOPHOSPHAMIDE (CYTOXAN)

This is the chemotherapy drug I mentioned in the Living section of this chapter. The most powerful medication of the group, Cytoxan has only anecdotal experiences suggesting its effectiveness in treating interstitial lung disease—although some researchers have documented a concurrent improvement in skin involvement. The good news: There is currently an NIH-funded Cytoxan study underway at multi-centers across the nation. This placebo-controlled study should provide the definitive answers we need about Cytoxan's effectiveness in treating scleroderma.

STEROIDS

Although quite useful for treating inflammation and overlap syndromes, steroids' placement in scleroderma's arsenal of disease-modifiying drugs remains extremely controversial. Some physicians wonder whether steroids have a place at all in the treatment of the disease.

The complexity of scleroderma makes it unlikely that there will ever be one particular treatment that will alter all the features of the disease. But with the increasing number of quality clinical trials, the likelihood of finding new therapies that will modify the disease outcome is more promising than ever before. You'll read more about clinical trials in Month 3.

Treating the Symptoms

DUE to scleroderma's complexity, successful treatment requires an individualized approach. Survival of scleroderma patients has greatly improved, mainly due to therapies focused on single organs. Besides the above-mentioned disease-modifying drugs, a plethora of drugs is available to relieve the symptoms of the disease. It's always best to speak to your physician about what would be the best course of treatment for you as an individual, but the following list will provide you with some basic information about what's currently available.

RENAL DISEASE

Early management of hypertension (high blood pressure):
- ACE inhibitors
- Angiotensin II inhibitors
- Calcium channel blockers

Management of renal failure:
- Dialysis

MUSCULOSKELETAL SYMPTOMS

Reduction of joint/tendon pain:
- NSAIDs (non-steroidal anti-inflammatory drugs)
- Analgesics
- Corticosteroids

Myositis:
- Steroids
- Immunosuppressive agents

GI SYMPTOMS

Acid reflux (heartburn):
- Antacids
- H-2 blockers
- Proton pump inhibitors

Bacterial overgrowth and malabsorption:
- Antibiotics

Motility issues (e.g., difficulty swallowing):

○ Prokinetic agents or GI stimulants

PULMONARY DISEASE

Pulmonary fibrosis:

○ Immunosuppressive agents

○ Steroids

Pulmonary hypertension:

○ Oxygen treatment

○ Prostacylin (inhaled, IV, or tablet form)

○ Endothelin antagonists

CARDIOVASCULAR DISEASE

Pericarditis:

○ NSAIDs

○ Corticosteroids

OVERLAP SYNDROMES

○ Steroids

○ Antimalarials

DEPRESSION

○ SSRIs (serotonin reuptake inhibitors)

○ Tricyclic antidepressants

○ Various newer agents

SKIN FIBROSIS

This is a highly individualized category. You must work closely with your physician to determine what treatment approach, if any, is best for you based upon the type and duration of your disease.

This list covers some of the more common symptoms of scleroderma. Obviously, other symptoms can occur, each with their own treatment strategies. I wish I could say there was one universal treatment strategy to treat your disease, but there isn't. (Many potential treatments are being studied, and there's great hope for the future.) Nevertheless, you do have options. Sometimes you and your physician will need to be creative. This may mean thinking "outside the box," to come up with just the right mix of medications for you. And if you're willing to be a bit experimental, some doctors can become very creative. For example, you and your physician might consider "off-label usage" of a medication. When a drug is approved by the FDA, it is approved only for the exact uses in which it was studied. But physicians often find a particular medication can provide benefits for other conditions as well. Off-label usage simply means the medication is being prescribed for something other than what it was initially tested and approved for. Before you and your doctor decide this type of treatment may be right for you, make sure you are aware of both the risks and benefits. I have taken off-label medications and have had very positive results. But that's me. Whatever decisions you make about your treatment, just make sure you're comfortable with the strategy and are willing to be a compliant patient. That's the most you can do to ensure the best results and outcome.

Dealing with the side effects

No matter how terrific a medication looks on paper, you're the one who has to decide how you feel while taking it. Does it control your symptoms but make your head so dizzy you can hardly walk? If so, this is not the right drug for you. You've learned by now that we all respond differently to medications. One person's euphoria may be another person's nightmare. If the side effects are making your life miserable, speak up. You do have options. Just because one medication doesn't work for you doesn't mean another won't. If your pain medication isn't doing the trick, this is not the time to be brave and "suck it up." You'll only be hurting yourself. Pain is not only physically draining—it's also emotionally draining. There's no need to suffer in silence when other solutions are out there. Just make sure you and your doctor are on the same page. You may find that you have very different treatment goals. He or she may be thinking long-term, while you're thinking short-term. Your goal may be just to get through your day without pain, while your doctor's goal may be to get you off pain medications as soon as possible. Whatever the differences are, make sure you are each aware of the other's reasoning. And if you don't get the results you need with your current mix of meds, try again. It may take some time, but eventually you'll find the right mix with the right results.

Be a cautious consumer

You are paying your doctor for his or her expertise and treatment recommendations, but the choice of what medications you take is yours. Learn as much as you can and try to have realistic expectations. Some medications take time to work and it may take a while before you notice their effects.

I've said this before, but I can't emphasize enough the importance of working closely with your physician to come up with a treatment plan that's right for you, and you only. Whether it be a "wait and watch" approach, or a "treat immediately" strategy, you need to feel comfortable with the plan and confident that it's the right one for you.

IN A SENTENCE:

> There is no cure for scleroderma, but there are disease-modifying drugs available, and medications to treat the symptoms.

WEEK **4**

Expect the Unexpected:
No Two Patients Are Alike

"WHY DOES Mary have skin involvement but I don't?"
"Why am I losing weight but Stacy's gaining weight?" "Why are
Joann's kidneys involved when my lungs are involved?" Sound
familiar? If you've been asking yourself these types of questions,
you're in good company. Unfortunately, you're unlikely to find
answers to these questions anytime soon—there simply aren't
any answers. Or answers that make sense, anyway.

As you learned in Day 2, this disease is unlike any other. And
because there are so many different types of scleroderma, your
disease manifestations may be unlike those of any other
patients you know or read about. This may make you feel more
alone with your disease. It shouldn't. It's completely normal for
you to have different symptoms and problems than other scleroderma patients. I had one doctor who coined my disease
"Gottesman's disease," as it was unlike any he had seen. That
variousness can be a challenge for doctors and patients alike.

Accepting the unexpected

Scleroderma has often been referred to as a disease characterized by exceptions. Just when you think you understand what's happening to your body, scleroderma throws you a curveball. It's times like these when you wish your disease had a more predictable path. Let's face it: There's nothing black and white about scleroderma. This is a gray disease. It varies both in severity and progression. When Joan was diagnosed with localized scleroderma, she expected the skin on her fingers and forearms to become tight, because this was how her particular disease manifested itself. What she didn't expect was that the skin under her armpits would tighten, as well. As with all new symptoms, a call to your doctor should be your first step. But do keep in mind that the new symptom you're experiencing, although not expected or classic textbook, may be completely normal for your particular type of disease. Among all the patients I've come in contact with over the years, I've never met a single person whose disease was like mine. I've even experienced symptoms that some of my doctors had never seen. Disconcerting? You bet. Especially during the first year, when everything was so new. But as time went on and unexpected symptoms would arise, I tried to deal with the unexpected from a different perspective. I realized how normal the unexpected was in a disease like scleroderma. If I was going to accept my disease, I realized, I was going to have to learn to live with the unexpected. But acceptance didn't happen overnight. It probably won't for you, either. Hopefully, as the weeks go on, the "expect the unexpected" mantra will slowly sink in. And remember, just because you expect the unexpected doesn't mean you'll never get frustrated or throw your hands in the air and say "What now?" To this day, I get frustrated by the exceptions to the disease. But now I know it's just another part of the journey.

There are many situations where you must prepare yourself for the unexpected

Living with a gray disease comes with its own set of challenges, such as not knowing what to expect, or always wondering what may happen next. How can you prepare yourself to handle some of these issues? The short answer is, you can't. But what you can do is learn about some of the more common situations that may challenge your sanity.

Several scenarios come to mind:

○ **Doctor appointments**—You may have a certain expectation of how you'd like a particular appointment to go. I know I do. Many times, on my appointments, I have a specific agenda in mind. But once you get to the appointment, you may find that your doctor has an entirely different agenda than yours. Perhaps he or she has some concerns about your latest lab results, or wants to talk to you about a new clinical trial. Now, the majority of your appointment time has to be spent on something entirely different than what you had anticipated. This happens all the time. And there are a few ways to handle it. Obviously, if you have an urgent medical need, it's up to you to make sure there's enough time to discuss it. If not, put your agenda in your back pocket and save it for next time. If you feel certain things on your agenda can't wait until the next appointment, kindly ask your doctor when a good time would be to phone him or her because you'll need a few extra minutes. Or perhaps you can e-mail your doctor—but check first. As common as e-mail is, plenty of physicians prefer not to communicate with their patients via e-mail. There's usually a solution to these types of problems; sometimes you just have to be creative to find it.

○ **Insurance companies**—I'm sure I don't need to say this, but: Insurance companies will become the bane of your existence. Consider the following scenario: You need to have a **magnetic resonance imaging (MRI)** test and your doctor wants it done immediately. You had the same test done several months ago and were told by your insurance company that you didn't need prior approval for the test. Great. You make your appointment for the next day, because after that, the next available appointment will be when your doctor's on vacation in Greece. You decide to play it safe and call your insurance company just to make sure you don't need approval. But this time, you talk to a different person, who says that you do indeed need prior approval and you must wait 48 hours to get it. You try to explain that you didn't need approval last time—why now? A word of caution:

Don't try to use logic when dealing with your insurance company. You'll only cause yourself more frustration and grief. Try to remain calm. And do not let them bully you. This scenario actually happened to me. But I was relentless with my insurance company. I told them this was the only time available to take the test and, like it or not, I needed approval by noon the next day. The next thing I knew, I was sitting in the hospital waiting room with a fully charged cell phone, praying the phone would ring before the nurse called my name for my test. And it did. I got my approval in the nick of time, but certainly not without a lot of angst. The lesson here is, just because a procedure worked one way last time doesn't mean it will work that way again. C'mon—it's your insurance company, remember?

○ **Drug reactions**—Your best friend was just prescribed a new pain medication and raved about the miracles of modern medicine. Not only was she pain-free for the first time in months, but she had literally no side effects from the medicine. You ask your doctor for the same medication, thrilled to know how well it works. Unfortunately, your scenario plays out a bit differently. What was a miracle drug for your best friend turns out to be your worst nightmare. Diarrhea, chills, headache, and a grogginess so severe you can't get out of bed. The lesson? What works for one person may not work for you. Everyone's body reacts differently to medications. Stop taking the medication and call your doctor as soon as possible.

○ **Disease manifestations**—Although some types of scleroderma may run a fairly predictable course, yours may not. It's best not to compare yourself to your mother's best friend's cousin who lives in Australia. Different person, different set of circumstances, different problems. Remember, you have a gray disease. Expect the unexpected.

○ **Your feelings**—I have a hunch these may surprise you the most. Mine sure did. Just when you think you've learned to accept your disease, something new comes along and throws you right back into a depression. This is normal. Don't be too hard on yourself. Just make sure you're able to work your way out again in a reasonable amount of time. Other feelings may pop up and surprise you as well.

That's okay, too. Whether you're feeling surprised, sad, fearful, or depressed, there's no need to fight the feelings. It's all part of the process of learning how to deal with the disease.

IN A SENTENCE:

> *Always be prepared for the unexpected in a disease like scleroderma and try not to compare yourself too much with other patients.*

learning

Don't Be Afraid to Ask for Help

DON'T BE afraid to ask for help. Sounds easy enough, right? Think again. This may be one of the hardest challenges you've faced yet. Especially if you're like me and are used to doing everything yourself. You've muddled through these last three weeks on your own and are now realizing you may need some help. Most people with a chronic disease do. But now you're asking yourself: Who do I turn to? How do I ask for it? How is it going to make me feel?

Self-reliance is a wonderful thing, but the reality is, we all need help at some point or other. Just because you need help doesn't mean you are a weak or needy person. In fact, I think you'll be quite surprised at how many people in your life are willing to help you. But don't ever assume people know that you need help. That's up to you. All you have to do is ask. Yep, it's that easy. The first step is recognizing you need help. The second step is getting past the uncomfortable feeling of asking for it.

Asking for help may be easier if you identify what type of help you need. Perhaps you're looking for emotional help or to enhance your spirituality. Maybe the thing you really need is physical help. Determining which type of help you need allows you to better focus on what resources are available to you. Say you're feeling too physically fatigued to clean your house. What options are available to you? If money's not an issue, you could hire a house cleaner. If that doesn't work, perhaps your spouse could pick up the slack. If you're without a spouse, maybe a close friend could help out. Or perhaps, when you're feeling better, you could trade chores with a neighbor. If you keep thinking along those lines, you're bound to come up with a solution. There's plenty of help out there. Sometimes you just have to think creatively to find the help you need.

Finding emotional help

TALK TO A MENTAL HEALTH PROFESSIONAL

Any physician will confirm this: Your mental health is just as important as your physical health. Most people I know with a chronic disease have some type of mental health professional on their team. You, too, may benefit from talking with a professional, whether a psychologist, psychiatrist, counselor, therapist, or social worker; just make sure you choose one you trust and with whom you feel comfortable. Don't be afraid of all the acronyms after their names (e.g., MSW, Ph.D, or LCSW) either. Sure, you want a qualified professional. But, more importantly, you need to feel that this person understands and respects you. As in any other relationship, you and your therapist must be a good fit. Some of you may feel there is a stigma attached to seeing a therapist or even that it's shameful. Look at it this way. If Tony Soprano can see a therapist, so can you. Acknowledging that you need help and seeking it out is one of the bravest things you can do. Ask your physician for a referral. You'll be glad you did.

LEANING ON YOUR SPOUSE, FRIENDS, AND FAMILY

Sometimes, all you may need is the comfort of knowing that there is someone in your life who will be there for you when you need him or her. This is where your spouse, friends, and/or family come in. Don't underestimate the positive effect these people have on your well-being—if you let them. Try not to shut them out. Those closest to you often want to help but feel helpless as to what to do. Try letting them do things like driving you to an appointment, doing the dishes, or just listening to your feelings. You'd be surprised at how even the littlest bit of help can make a big difference in your life. And it probably makes those in your life feel good to help you. It's a win/win situation for everyone.

SUPPORT GROUPS: FRIEND OR FOE?

If you don't feel comfortable talking about your disease with those closest to you, or you feel they truly don't understand what you're going through, consider a support group. Most of the patients I interviewed for this book had joined a support group at one time or another during the course of their disease. For some, there's nothing more comfortable than surrounding themselves with others going through a similar experience. It can be a welcome relief to share stories, talk about common issues, and learn about new, potentially helpful treatments or doctors in your area. For some people, talking to strangers about something so intimate is easier than talking to their own family and friends. Here's where a support group can be a wonderful thing. But they're not for everybody. Revealing your feelings to a group of strangers can also be very intimidating. Only you can determine if it's right for you. If you decide you'd like to join one, or at the very least check one out, call your local chapter of the Scleroderma Foundation to find the group closest to you.

Finding spiritual help

You may feel as though you need more comfort, peace, and serenity in your life and are looking to become a more spiritual person. Although you'll learn more about spirituality in Month 5, a good place to start is in learning the difference between religion and spirituality. The terms *religion* and *spirituality* are often used interchangeably, but they actually have very different meanings. Spirituality is a personal search for meaning and connection with a higher power. A person can be spiritual without belonging to a religion or attending religious services. Religion, on the other hand, refers to an organization or institution with established rituals, beliefs, and practices involving a community of others who share the same beliefs. According to Gallup polls, 95 percent of Americans believe in God or a universal spirit. And an overwhelming 79 percent believe that faith helps people recover from illness.

WHERE TO FIND IT

How does one go about getting spiritual help? One place to start would be your church, temple, or mosque, if you belong to one. Make an appointment with your religious leader or try to attend religious services. Attending services regularly allows you to benefit from the companionship and support that comes from being a member of a community. If religion is not comfortable for you, you can still benefit from the positive effects of the social support that goes along with most religious or spiritual groups. Just make sure you're not looking for a miracle. The rewards of a spiritual practice are focused on the process, not the results.

Another way to enhance your spirituality is through prayer or meditation. People have been finding comfort, meaning, and inspiration in prayer for thousands of years. It is generally accepted that prayer helps us to cope and offers great comfort in times of need. Meditation is used by those seeking to attain a state of enlightenment, peace, or closeness with God. It involves using any number of awareness practices to focus and quiet the mind and body. But meditation is not for everyone. Some people find it difficult to be still long enough to learn or practice the techniques—myself included. But that doesn't mean you shouldn't try it.

My only advice would be to keep an open mind. And trust yourself. Just because your best friend has become a Hare Krishna doesn't mean you should, too. A spiritual journey is a very personal one. If you feel you will be better able to cope by becoming a more spiritual person, then, by all means, go for it. Remember, spirituality and prayer are free. You have nothing to lose.

Finding physical help

Is your fatigue so overwhelming on certain days that you can't get out of bed? Do you find yourself asking the person standing next to you in line at Starbucks to tie your shoe for you? Are you unable to work the long hours you once used to? If you answered yes to any of these questions, you need physical help. The easiest way to start finding the help you need is to make a list of all the different areas in your life where you need physical help. Then go back over it and make a list of all the people you think can potentially help you in each area. Say, for example, you're having a bad week and are unable to get to the market. Your spouse is out of town and your parents live in another state. What are your possibilities? Several come to mind. Try shopping online at one of the many grocery delivery sites now available. Don't have a computer? What about asking a neighbor to pick up a few things for you when he or she next goes out? Or what about calling a sibling or a close friend to do the shopping for you? The possibilities are endless.

FINDING SOLUTIONS TO COMMON PHYSICAL PROBLEMS

To help brainstorm different solutions to some issues that may come about, consider the following:

1. *Need to work fewer hours?* Ask if you can work part-time, or talk to your boss about job sharing. You can even hire a vocation rehabilitation counselor to help provide you with new job training if you find you're unable to work in your current position. This is the perfect solution for the office worker who is unable to work due to hand deformities.
2. *Too tired to get the dinner dishes done?* Enlist the kids. Even the littlest ones are capable of lending a hand. And often, happily so.
3. *Can't open jars, or button your clothes?* There are lots of easy-to-use products available for just these types of problems. Some of the products include easy-open pill bottle caps, jar grippers, even products to help dress yourself. Check out Independent Living Products at *www.ilp-online.com* or look in the back of an *Arthritis Today* issue. With a little research, you can find just about anything you need.

Helping yourself

Congratulations. You've admitted you can't do everything on your own and that you need a little help. Your life will become easier from this point forward. I promise. If you're still having problems getting the help you need, please call the Scleroderma Foundation. They will do everything they possibly can to help you get the help you need and deserve.

IN A SENTENCE:

> *Asking for help is one of the best things you can do for yourself.*

FIRST-MONTH MILESTONE

By the end of your first month, you have gained further knowledge and understanding of scleroderma, by

○ LEARNING ABOUT ALL THE DIFFERENT TESTS YOU MAY NEED TO TAKE AND THE IMPORTANCE OF EARLY TREATMENT AND INTERVENTION;

○ UNDERSTANDING THAT ALTHOUGH THERE IS NO CURE FOR YOUR DISEASE, THERE ARE MANY MEDICATIONS AVAILABLE TO TREAT THE SYMPTOMS OF SCLERODERMA;

○ REALIZING THAT EVERY SCLERODERMA PATIENT IS DIFFERENT; AND

○ ACCEPTING THAT IT'S OKAY TO ASK FOR HELP.

The Doctor-Patient Relationship

AS YOU learned in Day 5, finding a good doctor to treat your disease is essential to your long-term health and well-being. By now, you've hopefully found a board-certified physician and feel confident in his or her ability to listen to your needs, as well as successfully treat your disease. The hard part is over. Or is it? Now comes the trickier part: how to successfully develop a positive and long-lasting relationship with your doctor. Sounds easy enough, right? Not necessarily. Due to the enormity of the power imbalance, there are few relationships as complex as the doctor-patient relationship. Over the years, the doctor-patient relationship has been defined as a relationship founded in trust. A patient will often reveal the most intimate details about his or her health and in turn, the doctor agrees to honor that trust and to become the patient's advocate. This is the foundation of the profession. It represents the expectation of how doctors and patients are supposed to behave toward one another. But this fiduciary relationship doesn't take into account the reality of each of these roles. The simple fact of being the patient defines your role as one of both vulnerability and dependency. The doctor's role, on the other hand, is defined by power and authority.

And because your roles are defined prior to entering the relationship, this power imbalance begins almost as soon as you establish the relationship. However, the presence of this power imbalance doesn't mean you need to lose sight of what you need out of the relationship. Remember, this is supposed to be a partnership. Let's talk about how to redefine your roles and expectations to create a mutually beneficial relationship between you and your doctor.

Developing a partnership

Having a chronic illness means you may require years of continual care, and your relationship with your doctor greatly influences your ability to make wise health care decisions along the way. A successful doctor-patient relationship should be defined by trust, confidentiality, and compassion. But this dynamic doesn't happen overnight. A good partnership, like any relationship, takes time to create. In an age when the average office visit lasts approximately 16 minutes, you must use your time extremely well. Let's take a look at what it takes to develop a long-lasting partnership with your doctor.

- ○ **Good communication is key.** The key to any successful relationship is good communication. Both you and your doctor must make an effort to talk openly and honestly about all aspects of your care. If you cannot communicate your needs and concerns for fear of how your doctor may react, you need to let your doctor know how you're feeling. Many people find it difficult to discuss sensitive subjects with their doctor; if this is the case for you, rest assured your doctor has probably heard it before. Remember, he or she can't treat a problem if he or she doesn't know it exists. Obviously, if your physician continually responds to your needs with rejection or impatience, find a new doctor.
- ○ **Make sure you have common goals.** Misunderstandings between a doctor and patient can arise from false expectations of what each can and should be doing. When a physician's goals aren't met, that physician is apt to label his patient as difficult. But you have goals, too. Make sure you both have the same agenda at each appointment. If your agenda is to completely eliminate your

What Kind of Patient Are You?

DOCTORS know they hold the power, and this can feel incredibly intimidating for the patient. But just because they're wearing the white coats doesn't mean the doctors get to make all the decisions. The doctor has as much power as you're willing to give. You, the consumer, are paying your doctor for his or her knowledge and expertise. It's up to you to decide what to do with that knowledge. To help you decide what kind of patient you are, here are some questions you might want to ask yourself:

1. *How much information are you comfortable receiving?* Are you the type of person who needs a lot of details in order to process the information you receive from your doctor, or are you the type who goes on information overload when presented with too many details? Don't be afraid to tell your doctor exactly how much, or how little, information you want.

2. *How involved do you want to be in the decision-making process?* There are those patients who would rather leave most decisions up to the doctor, and there are those who like to be presented with all the options and make the decision themselves. As you've read earlier, I'm a big advocate of patients taking an active role in their own care. In fact, chances are your doctor will be happy to know you're interested in taking an active role in your health care, as well. This role may not feel right for everybody, though; only you can decide what role you're willing to play. But your ultimate goal should be to establish a partnership with your physician—and this means becoming involved in the decision-making process.

3. *Are you looking for sympathy, support, or sound advice?* You probably chose your physician based on both his or her experience with sclerodema and his or her personality type. But now, you must evaluate exactly what you need out of the relationship. Obviously, you want your doctor to be both compassionate and sympathetic. Your main goal, though, should be to obtain sound medical advice. If your doctor's delivery of medical information leaves something to be desired, that's okay—as long as he or she is not rude and dismissive. If you're looking for more sympathy and support but feel confident in your doctor's knowledge and ability, you may want to think about adding a mental health professional to your medical team, if you haven't done so already. This way, you'll have someone else to talk to about your feelings and won't feel as disappointed when your physician doesn't meet all of your emotional needs.

pain, but your doctor's agenda is to help you learn symptom management, you're headed for trouble. Be honest with your physician about what your expectations are. And be honest with yourself, too.

○ **Learn how to resolve conflict.** Even the best relationships can have problems from time to time. If you've been pleased with your physician overall, it's worth the effort to try to resolve the conflict. Having an established relationship is worth a lot these days and working through the problem is often preferable to starting over with another doctor. Resolving the conflict requires talking openly and honestly about the problem. The solution may be something as simple as changing a tone of voice, or as complex as an entire overhaul of your latest treatment plan. Whatever it is, make sure you have reasonable expectations of the outcome. Ongoing conflict, on the other hand, should be examined more closely. If you find your needs just aren't being met, then it's time to search for a new doctor.

Patient expectations

We all have expectations of what our doctor should provide. As a patient, you should expect the following from your physician:

1. **A clear explanation of your illness and proposed treatment plan.** Never leave your doctor's office without a clear understanding of what your disease is about. You should also understand how it affects your body, your lifestyle, and your long-term health. You should also understand your treatment plan. Make sure to ask the following questions: Why was this particular treatment prescribed for me? What other options are there? How will this affect me in my day-to-day life?

2. **Confidentiality.** Trust is the glue of the doctor-patient relationship. Confidentiality is a key element of that trust.

3. **To be able to ask questions and receive understandable answers.** The language of medicine can get awfully complicated. Sometimes, your doctor may forget that you didn't go to medical school. When you don't understand something, ask your doctor to explain it in lay terms. And if you still don't understand, try rephrasing your questions until you receive a satisfactory answer.

4. ***Not to feel rushed.*** It's not your fault if your physician is running behind schedule. You deserve just as much time as the next patient. Don't let your physician take out his or her time frustrations during your appointment time. You pay for that time and are entitled to every minute of it.

5. ***To have your phone calls returned.*** And returned in a reasonable amount of time. Unfortunately, that phrase is open to interpretation. Remember, though: It's not up to your doctor to evaluate the importance of your phone call; it is your doctor's responsibility to return it. The reality is, however, that things do come up and your doctor may truly be unable to get back to you the same day. If that's the case, then it's not unreasonable to expect a phone call from his office staff asking if they can help you in any way and letting you know exactly when your doctor will be returning your phone call.

6. ***That your doctor knows his or her own limitations.*** If your physician reaches the limits of his or her knowledge and expertise, he or she should refer you to a specialist. Some of the physicians I've admired most have been the ones who recognize their own limitations.

7. ***To be able to comfortably disagree.*** Let's face it: There will be times when you and your physician won't be seeing eye to eye. And when you don't agree with something your doctor has said or done, you need to feel comfortable about speaking up. It's okay to disagree. Just make sure you're being reasonable instead of antagonistic.

8. ***To receive a thorough explanation of medications prescribed.*** This includes risks, benefits, drug interactions, and any known side effects. You should also know what the medication is for and for how long you will need to take it.

9. ***To be treated with courtesy and respect.*** Physicians are not always the best communicators and can often (intentionally or unintentionally) appear to be patronizing and arrogant. Don't accept this behavior. You deserve to be treated with respect and consideration.

10. ***To be able to get a second opinion.*** Some doctors may feel threatened by this, but a knowledgeable doctor won't. It's your body and your life. You have the right to get another opinion. Just make sure your insurance company will pay for it!

11. ***To have your emotional concerns addressed.*** Your doctor doesn't have to be your therapist, but he or she should provide a certain amount of empathy and compassion for your fears and concerns.

12. *To have your physician be your advocate.* It is not unreasonable to expect your physician to fill out disability forms, medication-related insurance forms, and any other information relating to your health and well-being. This is a partnership, remember?

13. *To not be afraid to ask a "dumb" question.* There is no such thing.

Doctor expectations

Turnabout is fair play. Your physician has expectations of you, as well. Your doctor expects the following from you:

1. *Come to the appointment prepared.* If you have many things you need to discuss with the doctor, it may be helpful to prepare a well-organized list of symptoms, problems, and concerns beforehand. This allows you to maximize your time with your doctor, and your doctor will truly appreciate your preparedness. Remember also to bring in a list of all your current medications and dosages; don't forget to mention any vitamins and/or alternative treatments you may also be taking.

2. *Be able to present a detailed past medical history of you and your family.* To the best of your ability, you need to be able to talk about your own past medical history, as well as your family's. This may include siblings, parents, and grandparents. If you need to show any past medical records, make sure to bring them with you to your appointment. A detail that seems insignificant to you may be just the piece of information your doctor needs to connect the dots.

3. *Be honest and straightforward.* This means being able to discuss not only detailed symptoms of your illness, but lifestyle issues as well. If you smoke, eat ice cream for every meal, or have never seen the inside of a gym, that's okay. Your doctor is there to help you, not judge you. As I mentioned earlier, your doctor can't treat a problem if he or she doesn't know it exists.

4. *Be a compliant patient.* If you don't intend to take a prescribed medication, say so. Your treatment is only as effective as you're willing to make it.

5. ***Actively listen to your doctor's medical advice.*** If you find your anxiety during your appointments is preventing you from hearing what your doctor is saying, bring along someone you trust to listen for you. It's always nice to have another pair of ears to hear the important details you may be missing. Another option may be to try to write down what the doctor says. Even under the best of circumstances, you may not remember everything you need to. But if you make a habit of taking notes, at least you'll have something tangible to go back to later on.

6. ***Take some responsibility for your own health care.*** This means not only being a compliant patient but also taking an active role in your health care. You should make every effort to understand your disease as best you can. And learn about your treatment, too.

7. ***Ask for clarification.*** If you don't understand something, make sure you speak up. Your doctor will assume you understand unless you tell him or her differently.

8. ***Address your main concerns early on in the appointment.*** Don't wait until the last minute of your appointment to bring up a new symptom or a problem you're having with a new medication. Begin your appointment with your most important concern. There's nothing more frustrating then getting to the end of the appointment only to realize you've forgotten to bring up your most important issue.

9. ***Don't expect an instant cure.*** And, don't make unrealistic demands. We all have high expectations of our physicians, but let's try not to forget: They're human, too.

Moving forward

In an era when doctor-shopping is as common as grocery shopping, it can be difficult to know the best way to establish a long-lasting doctor-patient relationship. Far too often, doctors are too quick to label their patients as demanding, noncompliant, or self-destructive, and patients are just as quick to label their doctors as arrogant, patronizing, and condescending. And all this occurs before they've even had time to get to know each other. It takes time to develop a satisfactory partnership with your doctor and it requires a commitment of honesty and respect from both parties. But once you've made that commitment, you'll be quite happy you took the time and made the effort to do so. Remember, your long-term health depends on it.

IN A SENTENCE:

A successful doctor-patient relationship involves open and honest communication, shared goals, and a strong belief in the value of developing a long-term partnership in your health care.

learning

Your Rights as a Patient

EVER WONDER what happens if your doctor refuses to provide you with a copy of your own medical records? Or how to go about finding out if your physician has ever had complaints filed against him or her? And what about the Hippocratic oath? Sure, you've heard of it, but what obligations does a physician have under today's version of the Hippocratic oath? If you've ever asked yourself any of these questions, or wondered about what your rights are as a patient, here's your chance to find out. Welcome to "Patient's Rights 101."

"Above all, do no harm"

A good place to start would be with the Oath of Hippocrates—a.k.a. the Hippocratic oath. We've all heard of it, but what does it actually mean? And do physicians actually abide by the tenets of an oath written in 400 BC?

A BRIEF HISTORY

The Hippocratic oath, written around 400 BC, was created as an expression of medical values and has endured throughout centuries of change in Western medicine. The Hippocratic oath came to define the Western approach to medicine and was used as the essential expression of medical values well into the early nine-teenth century. It was temporarily abandoned when science-based medi-cine became the mainstay of medicine; however, it regained momentum once it became apparent that science-based medicine couldn't be the judge of ethical conduct. The classical oath was divided into three sections:

○ Obligations to the profession and to patients
○ Specific rules to be observed in the treatment of disease
○ Expectations regarding the personal conduct of the physician

THE ROLE OF THE HIPPOCRATIC OATH
IN CONTEMPORARY MEDICINE

You're probably wondering what relevance the Hippocratic oath has in today's medical world. After all, the doctor-patient relationship has dra-matically changed over the last 50 years, with patients now forming "part-nerships" with their physicians and becoming increasingly more involved in their own treatment decisions and long-term health care. But, interest-ingly enough, recent studies have shown that a majority of U.S. medical schools report using some version of the Hippocratic oath during the "White Coat," or graduation, ceremonies. The oaths of today have been sig-nificantly revised from the original, although they have retained a few sec-tions true to the original, such as a physician's obligations to patients, as well as some stipulations about the personal conduct and character of the physician. Unfortunately, though, a few notable points have been omitted in today's versions. They include the following:

○ The covenants of the gods (no surprise there)
○ Prohibitions on euthanasia and abortion (no surprise there, either)
○ Conduct with regard to sex with patients (hmmmm)
○ Personal accountability for one's judgment and actions (bigger hmmmm)

Given the many changes over the years, what accounts for the contin-ued use of the Hippocratic oath in contemporary medicine? Essentially, the role of the oath today is to demand that the medical profession view itself, first and foremost, as a moral enterprise. Today the meaning of the Hip-pocratic oath exists more in what it stands for than in what it actually says.

The oath and your physician

You're probably asking yourself what effect the Hippocratic oath has on your own physician. We patients just assume that our own physicians abide by a set of ethical codes—after all, ethics is what the entire medical profession is based on: Besides the oath taken at graduation, each state's medical board upholds a code of ethics. And the AMA has adopted principles of ethics defining honorable behavior. But the truth is, most oaths in today's world are administered by voluntary agencies. So, what happens if you feel your physician has behaved unethically? What recourse do you have? The good news is that regulatory agencies that oversee physicians take allegations of unethical or unprofessional conduct very seriously. The voluntary agency may expel the physician from its membership or more serious action may be taken against a physician's license to practice medicine. You'll learn more about this procedure later in the chapter. First, let's take a closer look at some of your basic rights as a patient.

A *patient's bill of rights*

As a patient, you are entitled to certain rights. And if you're like I was, you probably have no idea what they are. Those rights are listed in *A Patient's Bill of Rights,* a document adopted by the American Hospital Association (AHA) over 30 years ago. The AHA is a national organization that represents and serves all types of hospitals and health care networks, as well as their patients and communities. According to the AHA, its mission is "to advance the health of individuals and communities. AHA leads, represents and serves health care provider organizations that are accountable to the community and committed to health improvement."

The document lists more than 12 specific rights that can be exercised by the patient or on the patient's behalf. Let's take a look at some of the key issues listed in the document, to remind ourselves of the type of care we are entitled to from our health care providers. The document can be viewed in its entirety at *www.hospitalconnect.com.* Some of your rights include the following:

- *The right to considerate and respectful care*
- *The right to obtain understandable information concerning diagnosis, treatment, and prognosis*

❍ *The right to review the records pertaining to your medical care, except when restricted by law*

❍ *The right to ask about and be informed of the existence of business relationships among the hospital, educational institutions, or other health care providers that may influence your treatment and care*

❍ *The right to have an advance directive*

❍ *The right to make decisions about the plan of care prior to and during the course of treatment*

Frequently Asked Questions

AS you navigate your way through the medical system, you may stop to wonder from time to time, "What happens if . . . ? "Hopefully, you'll never need to learn the answers to some of these questions. But on the off chance that this information may one day come in handy, here are answers to some of the most commonly asked questions regarding your personal rights as a patient:

1. *How can I find out if a physician has had complaints filed against him/her in the past?* There are two ways:

   ❍ The Federation of State Medical Boards provides a service called DocInfo, which provides physician disciplinary information for a small fee. You can check out its website at *www.docinfo.org*.
   ❍ Go to your state's licensing board. Not all states will provide this information, though, and those that do may charge a small fee.

2. *How do I file a complaint against a physician?* Once it's been determined that your physician has behaved unethically or unprofessionally, you have several choices. You may choose to discuss your concerns directly with your physician or perhaps with another physician who works in the same office. I, personally, would take it a step further and contact my state's medical society or licensing board if I felt the conduct warranted some type of action. These organizations have the appropriate investigative bodies at the local level to review the

physician's conduct and to take appropriate disciplinary action against the physician's license if need be. To find contact information regarding state medical societies and licensing boards, go to the American Medical Assocation's (AMA) website at *www.ama-assn.org*.

3. *What if my complaint is against a hospital or health plan?* If your complaint is against a hospital, you can contact the AMA at *www.hospitalconnect.com* or the Joint Commission on Accreditation of Healthcare Organizations (JCAHO) at *www.jcaho.org*. If your complaint is related to a health plan or health care insurer, or if you're wondering who to turn to if your health plan refuses to pay your physician, you can contact either the Health Insurance of America at *www.hiaa.org* or the American Association of Health Plans at *www.aahp.org*. If your complaint is related to a non-physician health professional (dentist, nurse, podiatrist, etc.) you can contact the professional association representing that particular type of health care worker.

4. *Can my doctor refuse to provide me with a copy of my own medical records because of an unpaid bill?* According to the AMA, your medical records "should not be withheld because of an unpaid bill for medical services." But keep in mind it is not unreasonable for your physician's office to charge you a small fee for copying them. In addition, you may be wondering how long your physician must keep your medical records. The AMA specifies that "while physicians have an obligation to retain patient records," the exact amount of time is largely affected by state law. You can contact your state's licensing board to find out what the regulations are in your state.

5. *What can I do if I feel my physician is charging too much?* If you believe your physician is charging an illegal or excessive fee, you can contact the appropriate specialty society through the AMA to find out what the appropriate fees should be.

6. *My physician has moved; how can I locate him/her?* The AMA has a service called Doctor Finder which can be accessed through its website at *www.ama-assn.org*. You can search for physicians by name, location, or specialty.

You're the boss

Learning about your rights as a patient is a topic you probably never thought you'd have to consider. Now that you've had some experience in navigating your way through the medical system, you're probably realizing the importance of ascertaining some basic knowledge about your rights as a patient. Even if you never have to exercise those rights, it's nice to know they exist. And plenty of organizations are available to assist you in obtaining your rights, if necessary. Feel comfortable in using them if you find you have to. This is just one more positive step to take in empowering yourself as a patient. The good news? You actually have more control than you thought you did. And all this time, you thought your doctor was the boss.

IN A SENTENCE:

Learning about your rights as a patient is an ongoing educational process that's essential to both your physical and emotional well-being.

Clinical Trials

YOU'RE AT a point in your disease where you may be considering several different treatment options. But now you find out some of these treatments are available only through clinical trials. You've heard the term **clinical trial** before but aren't sure what it is or what it entails. Here's your chance to find out.

What is a clinical trial?

A clinical trial is a research study involving the active participation of people (volunteers) to test the safety and effectiveness of new medical treatments or new ways of using an existing treatment. The term *study* is used very loosely to refer to an analysis. A medication in a trial has originated in a research laboratory and is studied for up to ten years in test tubes and lab mice before being tested for safety and effectiveness in humans. Only the treatments with the most promising lab results are moved to clinical trials. For many patients, a clinical trial is an opportunity to gain access to a medication as much as five or six years before it becomes commercially available. Clinical trials are designed to answer five basic questions about what they're investigating:

1. Is the medication safe?
2. Is it effective?
3. What side effects does it produce?
4. What dosage is most effective?
5. Is it more effective than or equally as effective as other treatments on the market?

The gold standard

The gold standard for clinical trials is called a *randomized, double-blind, placebo-controlled* trial. Let's break that down in lay terms:

- *Randomized* means that the researchers assign the people involved in the trial, at random, to either the experimental group or the placebo group. This ensures that the study outcome isn't biased or influenced by preexisting differences among patients assigned to study groups.
- *Double-blind* means that neither the patients, nor the researchers know who is getting the actual medication and who is getting the placebo.
- A *placebo* refers to an inactive medication that has no treatment value.
- A *controlled trial* compares the effects of a treatment on two or more groups of people. The experimental group gets the active treatment being studied; the control group may get a different treatment or a placebo.

The study results must be "statistically significant"—meaning the analysis must show that the difference between the treatment group and the placebo group is large enough that it could not be due to chance. Amazingly enough, as many as 30 percent of participants taking a placebo report having positive effects; if the treatment studied does not have a better result than the placebo, it's considered ineffective. ⁕

Who pays for clinical trials?

In the United States, pharmaceutical and biotechnology companies sponsor most clinical trials of medical treatments. In 2002, these companies spent more than $10 billion on clinical research. In addition to these sponsors, federal agencies such as the National Institutes of Health (NIH), the Department of Defense, and the Department of Veterans Affairs also fund clinical trials. Each year, government and industry sponsor more than 80,000 trials, representing as many as 5,000 to 6,000 protocols. What is a protocol? A protocol is a study plan on which all clinical trials are based. It describes

- ○ who may participate in the trial;
- ○ the schedule of tests, procedures, medications, and dosages; and
- ○ the length of the study.

Clinical trial phases

There are four phases to a clinical trial, each with a different set of objectives and requirements.

- ○ **Phase I**—The drug is tested for the first time, in a small group (20 to 100) of healthy volunteers. The phase typically lasts up to one year and its primary purpose is to evaluate the drug's safety, determine a safe dosage range, and identify side effects. About 70 percent of investigational drugs pass this phase.
- ○ **Phase II**—The treatment is now given to a larger group of people (100 to 300) who actually have the disease or condition the medication is being tested for. This phase usually lasts from one to three years and is used to further evaluate the drug's safety and effectiveness. Only about one-third of tested drugs successfully complete this phase.
- ○ **Phase III**—This stage provides hard statistical facts about a drug. The drug is given to a much larger group of people (1,000 to 3,000) and lasts two to four years. This phase confirms the medication's effectiveness, monitors side effects, and compares the drug with other commonly used treatments. At this stage, researchers also compare the drug's safety and effectiveness in different subsets of patients (men vs. women, elderly vs. young, etc.). They also test different dosage levels to determine how much of the drug is needed to achieve the best possible effects with the fewest side effects. About 70 to 90 percent of the drugs successfully pass this phase. Once this phase is complete, a pharmaceutical company can request FDA approval to begin marketing the drug.

○ **Phase IV**—This is referred to as the post-marketing phase. It involves several thousand patients and often lasts two to ten years. After a company has received FDA approval to market a drug, it will conduct this phase to uncover additional information about a new treatment, such as

  ○ what is the long-term safety and effectiveness of the drug?
  ○ what impact does it have on improving patients' day-to-day lives?
  ○ when do physicians prescribe this treatment versus similar treatments?
  ○ how does this treatment compare to similar treatments?

The results are used to further identify the drug's risks, benefits, and optimal use.

The FDA

The Food and Drug Administration (FDA) plays an important role in the clinical trial process. Not only does the FDA decide whether to give a new drug its stamp of approval and allow the drug to be marketed; the FDA also reviews study protocols and study results. It routinely sends inspectors to research centers to make sure that investigators are following the study protocol, treating the volunteers well, and following standard operating procedures for conducting research. FDA regulations also require Institutional Review Board (IRB) approval before a clinical trial can begin. An IRB is an independent committee, made up of physicians, statisticians, community advocates, and others, that evaluates a particular clinical trial. The IRB ensures that a clinical trial is ethical and that the rights of the study participants are protected. Before a clinical trial can begin, the IRB must do a risk/benefit assessment. Its goal is to make sure the level of risks involved in the clinical trial doesn't outweigh the potential benefits. The clinical trial participants can contact the IRB at any time to discuss any concerns they may have about their safety and protection.

Who participates in clinical trials?

All clinical trials have guidelines about who can participate. A participant must qualify for the study he or she is interested in being involved in. The criteria for participation are based on age, gender, the type and stage of a disease, previous treatment history, and other medical conditions. Some clinical trials need healthy participants; others need patients with the medical condition to be studied in the trial. The criteria used to determine qualification for a research study are there to keep participants safe, as well as to ensure that the researchers will be able to answer the questions they plan to study. The reality of a clinical trial is that it is designed to answer a scientific question, not to provide medical treatment. When considering participating in a clinical trial, you'll need to understand the difference between research and medical treatment. You'll learn more about whether a clinical trial is right for you in the Learning section of this chapter.

The Scleroderma Clinical Trials Consortium

As you learned earlier, there are no proven therapies to modify the course of scleroderma. And unfortunately, well-designed, randomized, controlled trials of adequate size and duration have been lacking. According to some of the top scleroderma researchers nationwide, the impediments to drug developments in scleroderma include

- ○ a low level of interest from the pharmaceutical industry;
- ○ incomplete understanding of the **pathogenesis** of scleroderma;
- ○ the absence of uniform and agreed-upon standards for design and conduct of clinical trials; and
- ○ the fact that scleroderma is an uncommon disease, which makes patient selection for trials very difficult.

The good news? As researchers' understanding of the disease process increases, new opportunities will be presented. Although the challenges of scleroderma clinical researchers are many, there is hope. The Scleroderma Clinical Trials Consortium (SCTC) is a charitable nonprofit organization dedicated to finding better treatment for scleroderma. The SCTC was started in 1994 with a handful of members and has grown to an international membership with over 50 centers in the United States, Canada, the United Kingdom, and Europe. Members of the SCTC have organized clinical trials on their own, with funding from organizations like the Scleroderma Foundation, the FDA, and the NIH. Not only are members studying medications currently on the market but not approved for scleroderma; they also support research to establish standard outcome measures for the trials, so that the results can be compared over time and with different patient groups.

The current clinical trials endorsed by the SCTC are listed on its website at *www.sctc-online.org.* You can also find lists of member institutions, clinical investigators, and study investigators, as well. If you're interested in participating in any of the trials, or would like additional information, you can contact the study coordinator at the number posted.

The bottom line

Clinical trials are essential to medical progress. New medical treatments must be proven safe and effective before the FDA can allow them to be used in the United States. The good news is that volunteers in clinical trials usually receive state-of-the-art care from physicians considered to be leaders in their field. And for some patients, the greatest benefit of a clinical trial is that it offers them hope. But the choice to participate should be given very careful consideration and should only be made after reviewing all the risks and the benefits involved. Although there is a limited pool of patients to draw upon with a disease like scleroderma, organizations like the SCTC are making it possible to further develop investigational therapies, bringing hope to scleroderma patients worldwide. For more information on clinical trials, you can visit *www.centerwatch.com,* an information source for the clinical trials industry, or *www.clinicaltrials.gov,* a website sponsored by the federal government.

IN A SENTENCE:

If you decide to participate in a clinical trial, you must understand the clinical trial process.

learning

Is a Clinical Trial Right for You?

CHOOSING TO participate in a clinical trial is a very important personal decision. In fact, only about 2 percent of the American population actually gets involved in clinical research each year. For some participants, getting involved in a clinical trial offers hope and a way to access investigational drugs that may be their only chance of survival. For others, their reason for participation may be as simple as not having medical insurance and needing help covering medical costs. According to a 2000 CenterWatch survey of 1,050 study volunteers, the following reasons were given as to why they participated in a clinical trial:

REASON	PERCENTAGE
Find relief or a cure	60%
Help advance science	23%
Earn extra money	11%
Receive better medical care	6%

There are even some people who make a profession out of being clinical trial volunteers. In deciding whether a clinical trial is the right choice for you, there are many things to consider.

Factors to consider before participating

All clinical trials carry some degree of risk. Before we talk about what questions you'll need answered before considering participation, let's take a look at some of the basic risks and benefits you need to be aware of:

RISKS

❍ The treatment may not be effective for you (i.e., you may receive the placebo). You may be trading a known treatment for an unknown treatment that has no benefits to your health.

❍ There may be unpleasant or very serious side effects to the treatment.

❍ The clinical trial protocol may require a big time commitment from you, including multiple trips to the study site, hospital stays, medical procedures, and complex dosage requirements. The trial can last anywhere from one month up to several years.

BENEFITS

❍ Participating in a clinical trial allows you to play an active role in your medical care.

❍ You can gain access to a new treatment long before it is commercially available.

❍ A clinical trial may give you access to expert medical care at leading institutions you wouldn't normally have access to.

❍ Your medical care is free during the trial.

❍ From an altruistic viewpoint, you'll be contributing to medical research and helping to advance science.

But that's not all you need to consider. You must do your homework.

YOU MUST GATHER OBJECTIVE ANSWERS
TO THE FOLLOWING QUESTIONS:

1. What is the main purpose of the study?

2. Who is sponsoring the study?

3. Who is participating in the study?

4. What are the eligibility requirements?

5. How long will the trial last?

6. What do researchers already know about the drug and what other studies have been done?

7. Where is the study being conducted? Multiple sites?

8. Does the study involve a placebo and, if so, what are my chances of getting a placebo?

9. What are the side effects of the drug?

10. How do the long-term risks and side effects compare with my current treatment?

11. What kinds of tests and procedures are involved?

12. Will I be reimbursed for any out-of-pocket expenses?

13. Will hospitalization be required?

14. What type of long-term follow-up is involved in the study?

15. How will I know if the treatment is working?

16. What happens if I quit the study?

17. What if I get the placebo but need the actual drug?

18. Will the results of the trial be provided to me?

19. Who is in charge of my safety?

20. How much of my time will this take?

21. How will this affect my daily life?

22. For what percentage of people will the drug be effective?

It is the principal study investigator's responsibility to give you enough time to ask all your questions, as well as to make sure you understand the answers. If you don't get the answers you need the first time around, ask again. This is a big decision. Take your time and consider the impact this study will have not only on your overall health but in your daily life, as well.

Factors that may exclude you from participation

All clinical trials have requirements that might render you ineligible for participation. Many people may be deemed ineligible just by a prescreening over the telephone. Some of the most common factors that may disqualify you from a particular study include

- ○ participation in another clinical trial within the last 30 days
- ○ drug use or alcohol abuse
- ○ pregnancy
- ○ allergy to ingredients in the study drug
- ○ refusal to use birth control (women only)
- ○ certain disease processes you may already have, such as kidney failure or heart disease
- ○ preexisting health conditions
- ○ current medications you are using

In some cases, researchers may modify eligibility requirements after a trial has begun. Perhaps there may be new findings about the investigational drug or too few patients have enrolled. If you were originally ineligible when the trial first began, you may want to periodically check in with the researchers to see if the requirements have changed and you would now be eligible to join the trial.

Giving your informed consent

Informed consent is a process that allows you to learn all the facts about a clinical trial before deciding whether or not to participate. Make sure to bring along the questions listed in the box above. This is the time to get your answers. Even though your signature is needed, the informed consent process is more about listening to the researchers explain the details of the study, getting your questions answered, and reading information about the clinical trial than actually signing a piece of a paper. However, the FDA does require that every adult volunteer agree to the terms *in writing* before they can enroll in a clinical trial. Informed consent insists on three basic things:

1. The volunteers are told everything about the study, including the risks.
2. The information is easy to understand.
3. The volunteers who agree to participate do so voluntarily, rather than being pressured or swayed into it.

The investigators or the study coordinator should review the consent form document with you, page by page. It should include details about the study, its purpose, duration, required procedures, key contacts, and potential risks. Some informed consents also contain a list of circumstances under which the investigator may terminate a volunteer's participation. Also included are the reasons for various research steps, potential benefits, and other treatment options. Do not sign it until you thoroughly understand what you are signing. If you feel the need, you may decide to take it home and have someone else read it as well. The consent form is essentially a contract between you and the research investigators—although not a contract in the literal sense, as the participant may withdraw from the trial at any time. Your signature represents neither a legal nor ethical obligation for you to participate. It merely indicates your permission to volunteer in the study for as long as you choose. Always remember: Even though you've signed an informed consent, you can leave the trial at any time. If you do decide to leave the trial, let the research team know that you are leaving and why.

The responsibilities you assume by signing an informed consent

Although you assume no legal obligations by signing an informed consent, it is your responsibility to be as honest as possible and to comply with the rules of the clinical trial. Dishonesty not only invalidates the study results but can potentially be dangerous to your health. This means

○ never lie to qualify for a clinical trial, no matter now badly you want to participate, and

○ always follow the study protocol. If you're instructed not to drink alcohol during the trial but decide to do so anyway, you're not only putting yourself at risk but also potentially invalidating the results of the trial.

Factors that may make you decide to leave the clinical trial

1. You received the placebo instead of the actual drug.
2. You can't handle the side effects and are concerned about the long-term risks.
3. You have unrealistic expectations of the outcome of the clinical trial.
4. You decide that another, already available treatment would be better for you.
5. The trial is inconvenient and too time-consuming for your lifestyle.
6. You're afraid of losing access to the medication once the trial is over.

Most volunteers have a positive experience

Although researchers have always had difficulty recruiting patients, a recent study published in the *Archives of Internal Medicine* shows the problem is worsening. It was found that not only are Americans deeply suspicious of medical research but there seems to be a limited pool of patients to draw upon, due to the rarity of some of the disorders the investigational drugs are being tested for. Another problem seems to be incredibly strict eligibility requirements. But, here's the good news: The volunteers who actually *do* participate in clinical trials all have positive experiences. Most volunteers report receiving very good quality care and note the high level of professionalism among the study staff. Most volunteers said they would participate again.

How do scleroderma patients feel about clinical trials?

Scleroderma patients seem to feel similarly positive. Of those interviewed who have participated in a clinical trial, the majority would happily participate again. One patient claimed that the clinical trial was a good experience but was very disappointed when the drug wasn't approved. She said she was treated very nicely throughout the entire trial and never experienced any bad side effects. Another patient said that being in a clinical trial gave her a sense of control over her disease and made her feel like she was being very aggressive in fighting scleroderma. Her only disappointment was that the trial was deemed inconclusive even though she felt that the drug had helped her.

Each person's experience in a clinical trial is unique; no two people, even with the same diagnosis, will react in the same way to a particular drug. Participating in a clinical trial is a big decision. You must not only be aware of the clinical trial process but also of how it will impact your daily life. Make sure you understand your rights as a volunteer and have a thorough knowledge of the trial's risks and benefits. Maybe the reason you initially enrolled is not the same reason you choose to remain. Regardless, the choice to participate remains yours and yours only.

IN A SENTENCE:

> *Clinical trials offer hope to many scleroderma patients but should only be considered after you thoroughly investigate whether the benefits of the trial outweigh the risks.*

living

What About Your Job?

WELCOME TO your latest worry: your job (as if you didn't have enough to worry about). For most people, their job represents financial security. For others, it represents who they are as a person. Sometimes a person's entire identity is wrapped up in this one particular area of life. This situation is especially true for doctors, police officers, attorneys, firefighters, actors, entrepreneurs, and other professionals. So it's no wonder that when your own job comes into question, your entire life can be turned upside down in a flash. Not only is your financial security at risk; your personal identity may come into question as well. Linda was a police officer when she was diagnosed. She had been feeling a bit fatigued but attributed it to her age and her job. Imagine her surprise when she was diagnosed from a routine dental problem. She was completely blindsided. Unfortunately, she went into kidney failure soon after and lost 20 pounds. She thought she was going to die. It was then that she realized her whole life was about to change. Due to the stress and physicality of her work, she had to quit her job. Then depression set in and didn't let up for six months. Police work had been her world and she loved her job. But when faced with the harsh reality of having to choose between saving her life or continuing her work as a police officer, she made the obvious decision. Nevertheless, mentally, it was brutal for her. She said, "I have never been so scared in my whole life. This, coming from a police officer!" Obviously, not all work-related situations are as black and white. If Linda's life had not been at stake, her decision may not have been so easy. Your own situation, for that matter, may not be so cut-and-dried. And that can make for some tough decision-making.

There is no easy answer

It's one thing to be forced to make a decision. It's another when your situation isn't as clear-cut. When I was first diagnosed, I was working for Bristol-Myers Squibb. Although I never considered my job to be particularly stressful, it was a fairly physical one. I often saw as many as 10 to 12 doctors in a day, and that meant a lot of driving and a lot of schlepping. Before I knew what was wrong with me, I remember feeling so overwhelmingly fatigued during the day that I often found myself sitting down in the doctor's waiting room, unable to get up. And the fatigue only got worse. After my official diagnosis, I continued working as my condition worsened. The worse I felt, the harder I pushed. I'd go back and forth from one exhausting situation to another. (Did I mention I also had twin toddlers at home to take care of? Talk about exhaustion!) Not one to give up easily, I continued like this for quite some time. Finally, my doctor looked at me one day and said, "Karen, something's got to give." Being the smart-ass that I am, I replied, "Okay, okay . . . I'll give up the disease." Not finding much humor in my response, he sat me down with a very serious look on his face and painted what I considered a very bleak picture of what could happen to me. Unfortunately, he turned out to be right. Shortly after his lecture, my lungs quickly deteriorated and I had to begin chemotherapy treatments. Only then did I realize I had to quit my job. The good news for me was that my job was only a means to an end. It never defined who I was or how I felt about myself. And although I felt like I was giving up a lot at the time, I see now that I didn't have a choice. There was no way I'd be able to take care of myself and my family if I didn't take care of my own health first. When all is said and done, your health should always come first, even if that means making some difficult choices. You'll read more about this in the Learning section of Month 10.

Important issues to consider

If you find yourself faced with work dilemmas, don't despair. You'll learn about the Social Security disability process in the Learning section of this chapter, and other options may be available to you as well. First, though, let's talk about some important issues you must take into account before you consider changing or leaving your current job situation.

❍ *Health insurance*—If you're thinking about quitting your job and are currently receiving health insurance benefits from your employer, you must think ahead. Gone are your carefree days of quit now and worry later. If you leave or lose your job, you are eligible for COBRA insurance for an additional 18 months (sometimes longer, depending on the circumstances). But unfortunately, you have to pay the insurance premiums yourself. If you're leaving your job for another one, you must find out about your new health insurance plan ahead of time. Many policies have preexisting condition clauses that may prohibit coverage on your disease for 3 to 12 months. If you're married, another option would be to get coverage from your spouse's policy. But again, don't forget to look into the preexisting condition clause of your new policy. It's up to you to find out exactly what your insurance policy will cover, as the rules can vary from state to state.

❍ *Financial security*—The reality of your situation may be that you just can't afford to quit your job right now. Or can you? You'll learn about disability and SSI insurance options available to you in the Learning section of this chapter; sometimes, though, you have to dig even deeper to find solutions. Especially if your health depends on it. If you're married and your spouse is working, try redoing your budget to see if you can both live on one income. You'd be surprised at how much you can save by reassessing your needs and making cutbacks. If you're single, one possible solution may be to take a temporary leave of absence from your job. Then, once your disease has stabilized, you can return to work when you're feeling healthier, both mentally and physically.

❍ *Personal identity*—If your self-worth is tied up in what you do for a living, you're in for a double whammy. Not only will you feel the financial loss, but you'll be reeling from a full-blown identity crisis too. And this crisis can lead to depression. This is the time to find other things in your life that make you feel good about yourself. Don't view this as a loss. Consider it an opportunity to explore other areas of your life that can provide a similar sense of self-worth. It may take some time, but after a while you'll find new doors opening for you that you never thought possible. All you have to do is knock.

Finding solutions

Finding a solution to your work-related problems might not be as hard as you think, especially if you've been working for your company for a long time. Most employers realize the value of good, loyal employees and are usually willing to work with them to accommodate their health needs. Consider the following options:

- O **Consider working part-time.** Cutting back on your hours may be all you need to do to get the extra rest you need. The cutback can be temporary or permanent, depending on your needs. My own employer was incredibly understanding of my health issues and allowed me to cut back on my hours for as long as I needed, to help me get back on my feet. Not all employers are this understanding, but you'll never know about yours until you ask.
- O **Try working from home.** These days, all you need is a computer and a phone to get your job done from just about anywhere. Working from home allows you to take the restful breaks you need in a more peaceful environment. If your employer doesn't want you away from the office every day, ask if you can work from home two to three days a week. It's a nice compromise for both parties.
- O **Consider job-sharing.** This is an ideal solution in theory but can be a bit tricky to implement. Not only do you have to find a compatible partner to work with, but also you have to make sure the whole process is not more trouble than it's worth. Although you're supposed to be working less, some overachievers try to cram a full week's worth of work into their shortened week, knowing they have less time to get it done. On the flip side, I know many people who have achieved ideal job-sharing partnerships and would never consider going back to working full-time.

○ **Take a leave of absence.** As I mentioned above, a leave of absence can be the perfect short-term solution to get you back on your feet. Talk to your employer about how much time he or she will allow you to take. You may be surprised at your employer's willingness to accommodate your needs during this time.

There are plenty of solutions to job-related problems if you look hard enough. Jobs come and go, but your health is here for the rest of your life. In your quest for the perfect solution, remember: Your health should always come first.

IN A SENTENCE:

As important as your job is to your well-being, your health should always come first.

learning

Surviving the Social Security Disability Process

YOU'RE AT a point in your disease where you're not able to work anymore. Or, you're not at that point yet, but you know you need to explore your options. It's time to learn about the various kinds of disability benefits available to you, but you don't know where to start. No one likes to think of themselves as disabled. But you're not alone. Your chances of becoming disabled before reaching retirement age are greater than you realize. Resources such as worker's compensation, disability insurance, and other personal means of support are also available to you, but this chapter will focus on Social Security disability benefits. Chances are, you have heard of Social Security disability benefits or Supplemental Security Income but haven't a clue as to what they are. The only thing you've heard about is how difficult it is to navigate the system. One scleroderma patient claimed that going through the Social Security disability process was actually worse than being diagnosed with the disease! But that's not always the case. Let's try to navigate through the process together so you don't have the same experience.

How is disability defined?

While other programs have different definitions for disability, it's important to understand how the Social Security Adminstration (SSA) defines disability. According to the federal Social Security Disability Act, disability is defined as an "inability to engage in any substantial gainful activity by reason of any medically determinable physical or mental impairment which can be expected to result in death or is expected to last for a continuous period of not less than 12 months." In lay terms, this means you will be considered disabled if you cannot do the work you did before and Social Security decides you cannot adjust to other work because of your medical condition. The step-by-step process used to determine if you are disabled involves five questions:

1. **Are you working?** If you're still working and making over $800 per month, you're generally not considered disabled.
2. **Is your condition "severe"?** Your claim will only be considered if your condition interferes with basic work-related activities.
3. **Is your condition found in the list of disabling impairments?** Social Security maintains a list of disabling impairments that automatically qualify you as being disabled. If your condition is not on its list, the condition must be considered of equal severity to those on the list for your claim to be considered.
4. **Can you do the work you did previously?** Social Security must determine whether the severity of your condition interferes with your ability to do the work you did previously. If the agency decides that it doesn't, your claim will be denied.
5. **Can you do any other type of work?** Your age, education, past work experience, and medical condition will be evaluated to determine if you are able to adjust to other work. If it's decided that you can't adjust to other work, your claim will be approved.

Now, before you move forward thinking this process is a piece of cake, let me warn you: It's not. In fact, the government makes this process extremely difficult. The complicated forms, the long waiting lines, and the general bureaucracy involved leave most people horribly frustrated or discouraged, and many give up. This is exactly the government's intention.

Legitimate claims are often denied at least once, sometimes twice or even more. This is completely normal. But here's a tip: Statistics clearly show that people who have representation (lawyers) win their benefits more often than those who apply on their own. Even though it may cost you a little bit more (although lawyers generally don't get paid unless you win your case), hiring an attorney is well worth it. Not only do attorneys have experience with these types of claims, but they have a much better understanding of the way Social Security works. Plus, who needs the extra headache? You have enough to deal with right now. Let someone else fight the government for you.

How to start the process

If you decide to apply on your own, you can begin the process at any Social Security office near you. You can file in person, on the phone, or by mail; Try to shorten the process by providing Social Security with the appropriate documents and medical evidence to support your claim. But before you begin, you should make sure you are even eligible for benefits. To qualify for Social Security benefits, you must have worked long enough and recently enough at a job that is covered under the provisions of the Social Security Act. To find out more specifics about eligibility, you can call the SSA at 800-772-1213 or go to its website at *www.ssa.gov*. But let me clarify one thing. Just because you qualify for disability *does not* mean your claim will be approved.

Once you've completed your application, it will be reviewed to make sure you meet the basic requirements for benefits. Afterward, it is sent to the Disability Determination Services (DDS) office in your state. The DDS will then determine whether you are disabled, based on the information provided.

If your claim is approved

Once a decision is made on your claim, a letter will be sent letting you know that your claim was approved. The letter will show the amount of your benefits and when the payments will start. Generally, your first benefits will be paid in the sixth full month after the date your disability began. For example, if Social Security determines your disability began on

January 1, your first payment will begin on July 1. The amount you receive will be based on your lifetime average earnings covered by Social Security. There are other details also factored into the amount you receive, such as other government benefits you may be receiving. You can find out more information about this or how this might affect your claim by checking the website.

In general, you will receive your benefits for as long as you are disabled. Your case will be reviewed periodically to determine whether you are still disabled. Two things can cause your benefits to be discontinued:

1. You're still working at a level that Social Security considers "substantial." "Substantial" is defined as average earnings of $800 or more per month.
2. Your medical condition has improved.

Frequently Asked Questions

○ *What is the difference between Social Security disability (SSD) benefits and Supplemental Security Income (SSI) benefits?* The medical requirements for disability are the same under both programs, but eligibility for SSD is based on prior work experience, and SSI benefits are made on the basis of financial need.

○ *Is my family entitled to Social Security benefits as well?* Only dependent children under 18 and those who still attend high school are eligible.

○ *If I'm a stay-at-home mom but I used to work, am I eligible to receive benefits?* Yes, if you were employed five out of the last ten years, in a postion that qualifies for benefits under agency rules, before you became disabled.

○ *What if I'm collecting early retirement?* Yes, you are still eligible, if it is determined that your disability began before you decided to retire.

○ *Can I still get Medicare if I'm disabled?* You will automatically be enrolled in Medicare after two years of receiving disability benefits.

○ *Can I receive benefits while I work?* Social Security provides many "work incentives" or "employment support" programs. Call your local Social Security office for more information.

If your claim is denied

Unfortunately, denial of claims occurs pretty commonly. As I mentioned earlier, many people are denied not only on their first application but on subsequent claims, as well. If this happens to you and you haven't hired an attorney yet, you might want to think about doing so now. Your chances of winning your claim on your second try are much greater with an experienced attorney handling your case. If you don't want to hire an attorney, you can appeal the claim yourself and have the Social Security office help you with the paperwork. But don't wait too long. You have only 60 days from when you received your denial to file your appeal.

Although the disability process can be both overwhelming and intimidating, it may be your only option. Make sure you've done your homework before you apply, to ensure you're familiar with the process. For many of you, the process may take quite a long time; others of you may win your cases immediately. But when you stop and ponder why it works one way for some and another way for others, remember one thing: You're dealing with the government—so don't expect answers anytime soon.

IN A SENTENCE:

> It's best to prepare yourself for a potentially lengthy and frustrating process when you apply for Social Security disability benefits.

MONTH **5**

living

Yoga, Herbs, Diet, and All the Rest

COMPLEMENTARY MEDICINE, alternative medicine, unconventional medicine, nonconventional, unproven . . . call it what you want. But there's a reason nearly half of all U.S. adults go outside the conventional health care system looking for answers. Welcome to the world of complementary and alternative medicine (CAM). It looks as if it's here to stay: Not only are conventionally trained physicians at some of the country's leading hospitals and research institutes studying herbs, acupuncture, tai chi, and whatnot, but the U.S. government has caught on, as well. In 1998, the National Institutes of Health turned its tiny Office of Alternative Medicine into a full-fledged federal agency called the National Center for Complementary and Alternative Medicine (NCCAM). Its tiny $2 million budget quickly rose to $100 million per year. Some of NCCAM's main ventures include projects such as assembling large clinical trials to assess the benefits of popular therapies like the supplement glucosamine, and looking into whether acupuncture can actually ease arthritis pain.

But there's a twist. Even though knowledge of CAM is on the rise among the government and patients alike, some doctors have yet to jump on the bandwagon. According to the Arthritis Foundation, nearly 70 percent of physicians don't discuss alternative therapies with their patients, mainly due to lack of knowledge. Besides, the Western approach to medicine has always been to recommend treatments that have been adequately tested in controlled trials. Most alternative therapies lack solid evidence to show that they are safe and effective. But this type of thinking is beginning to change. As patients begin to take a more active role in their health care, they're more willing to try complementary or alternative therapies to help gain some control over chronic ailments that have been unresponsive to conventional medicine. And doctors are beginning to listen. They're beginning to realize that some of these therapies, in conjunction with mainstream, modern medicine, can have a positive influence on overall health and well-being.

Which therapies are right for you? Meditation and yoga are accepted treatments for both stress and anxiety, and sometimes even pain. But what if you're considering some of the more popular therapies that claim to provide miracle "cures" or "natural" healing? Consider this: Besides being completely useless, some of these treatments can be downright dangerous. Remember, CAM can't replace proven treatments or cure your disease. Always be a cautious consumer. Familiarize yourself with the language of CAM, and learn the differences in their meanings.

Complementary vs. alternative vs. holistic vs. integrative medicine—what do they all mean?

The phrase *complementary and alternative medicine* covers a broad range of philosophies, approaches, and therapies. Before learning what those are, it's important to become comfortable with the industry lingo:

○ **Alternative medicine**—One of the most common terms used today to describe all types of unconventional therapies, it actually means "replacing" conventional treatments. A good example of using alternative medicine would be choosing to use an herb instead of a prescribed medication to treat your pain.

○ **Complementary medicine**—Complementary therapies are used "in conjunction with" or in support of mainstream medicine. Complementary medicine is used together with your prescribed treatment plan. One example would be using massage or aromatherapy along with your other prescribed therapies.

○ **Holistic medicine**—A philosophy of medicine that takes into account not only the physical aspects of the healing process but the mental, emotional, and spiritual aspects, as well.

○ **Integrative medicine**—A relatively new term in the medical world, it describes medical care that integrates complementary therapies with Western medicine.

○ **Western medicine**—Medical treatment and therapies taught in U.S. medical schools and used in most hospitals.

○ **Preventative medicine**—A philosophy of medicine in which a person is treated to prevent health problems before they arise, rather than treating the symptoms after a problem has occurred.

○ **Unconventional medicine**—Any type of treatment or therapy that doesn't fall within the scope of Western medicine.

How to get started

Now that you have a better understanding of the terminology, let's go further. You're interested in learning what's available to you but have no idea where to start. Specifically, you wonder what types of treatments are used for what ailments. But with all the advertising hype surrounding alternative treatments, how do you know what's really safe and effective? Needless to say, entire books have been written on this subject. If you're a novice, you might start the learning process by determining what your goals are. Ask yourself the following questions: Are you looking for a gentler form of exercise? Are you looking for ways to cope with your mental anxiety and stress? Are you looking for an herbal supplement to help you with your joint pain? Perhaps you're just interested in learning about ancient healing systems. Identifying what your needs are will help you focus your search in the right direction.

Be a Smart Scleroderma Patient and Consumer

AS A scleroderma patient, there are a few things you should be aware of before you begin. First, you should know that your immune system does not need to be improved. Many herbs touting miracle immune-boosting properties can actually make your symptoms worse. Your immune system is already overactive; you don't need any supplements to enhance it. Second, many herbs and over-the-counter medications can interact with some of the prescription drugs you're taking. They can even make your symptoms worse. Never take any herb, supplement, vitamin, or questionable remedy without checking with your physician or licensed practitioner first. But you knew that.

The NCCAM Complementary and Alternative Medicine categories—a broad overview

The NCCAM has classified complementary and alternative medicine into five distinct categories. If you're new to this territory, you'll find the categories a useful way to distinguish one therapy from another. Although some of the therapies may fall under more than one category, you'll find each listed only once. (Some of the more common therapies, such as massage or prayer, don't need any explanation.) If you'd like to learn more about a particular type of therapy, most have their own organizations, which can be found through a simple Internet search. The NCCAM categories are as follows:

1. ***Alternative medical systems***—These are healing systems based on their own theories of health, disease, and practice. Many were developed long before the availability of dependable drugs and surgery. Some of the oldest healing systems include the following:

   ❍ *Chinese medicine*—Originating some 2,000 years ago, it is best known in the United States for its acupuncture and herbal medicine. Its practice is based upon balancing the yin and yang—

interdependent but often opposing forces of nature. Also involved in this philosophy is a vital life energy called *qi* ("chee"). It is thought that when the flow of *qi* is blocked or is out of balance, illness occurs. Treatments are focused on helping you regain this balance by unblocking the flow of *qi* and strengthening the balance of yin and yang. This is done through the practices of acupuncture and acupressure. Chinese herbs play a key role as well. You'll learn more about these herbs in the Learning section of this chapter.

○ *Acupuncture*—Used by over 15 million Americans, acupuncture involves the practice of inserting very fine metal needles into the skin at specific sites in the body, to help manipulate your *qi*. Most commonly used to treat pain, acupuncture can also be used to treat a host of other conditions, such as nausea and digestive problems. In fact, my sister used it to help with her migraine pain and had great success.

○ *Acupressure*—This is much the same as acupuncture, but pressure is used instead of needles.

○ *Ayurveda*—This ancient healing tradition of India is perhaps the oldest of all medical systems. Its practices are noninvasive and focus on diet, exercise, moderation, and meditation. Its success depends on a person's willingness to commit to a pattern of healthy daily living. This usually involves a vegetarian-type diet, including herbs and supplements. Yoga and breathing exercises are also used to help balance energy. One of the most popular ayurvedic practitioners in the United States is Deepak Chopra.

Alternative systems that have developed in Western culture are the following:

○ *Homeopathic medicine*—Drawing on the theory that "like cures like," a homeopath gives patients tiny amounts of medicinal substances to cure the symptoms. Ironically, the same substance given in higher amounts would actually cause the same symptoms.

○ *Naturopathic medicine*—This focuses on the person rather than the disease; the main principles involve encouraging healthy living habits and allowing the body to heal itself through massage, exercise, and dietary modifications.

2. ***Mind-body interventions***—This category focuses on the ways in which emotional, mental, and physical factors interact and affect your health. The therapies help patients regain control over their lives by reducing pain, depression, and mental/emotional stress. Some of the therapies include

   - *Meditation*
   - *Aromatherapy*—Massage therapy with fragrant essential oils extracted from flowers, herbs, and fruits
   - *Hypnosis*
   - *Prayer*
   - *Gentle exercise techniques:* Yoga, tai chi, and qi gong (a self-healing art that combines movement and meditation)
   - *Biofeedback*—Shown to help relieve headaches, pain, and Raynaud's phenomenon, this therapy uses electronic monitors to teach you how to use your mind to affect different body systems
   - *Visualization*—Used mostly to help relieve stress and anxiety, this technique teaches you to use your imagination to attain relaxation and change behavior patterns

3. ***Biologically based therapies***—Often called nature's remedies, this category includes

   - *Herbs*
   - *Vitamins*
   - *Dietary supplements*

4. ***Manipulative and body-based methods***—Based on manipulation and movement, these practices include

   - *Massage*
   - *Reflexology*—A massage therapy that massages points mainly on the feet (hands and ears are used, too) that are believed to correlate to organs and other body parts.

○ *Chiropractic*—Also an alternative medical system, this therapy is used by more than 50 million Americans each year. It focuses on the manual adjustment of the spine to enhance bodily structure and function.

5. **Energy therapies**—This category of treatments uses biofield therapies and biomagnetic-based therapies to help many different musculoskeletal conditions. Some of the therapies include:

○ *Reiki*—A technique in which spiritual energy is channeled from the practitioner to the patient.
○ *Pulsed magnetic fields*—Not approved for use in the United States, this therapy involves sending a pulsed signal through an electromagnetic field to the area of the body being treated.

This list is only a broad overview of the most common complementary and alternative treatments available. Believe me, there are plenty more to be found. People seem willing to give anything, from bee venom to copper bracelets, a try these days. Now that you have a basic understanding of what some of these therapies involve, you can begin to do your own research on those you're most curious about. Keep in mind, there is no one type of therapy that is going to cure your scleroderma. And you may need to try quite a few different types before you find the right therapy to achieve your goal. As always, remember the cardinal rule: Make sure you discuss it with your physician first.

What about diet?

Fad diets. Elimination diets. Special diets. Fasting diets. Vegetarian diets. Vegan diets. Macrobiotic diets. Protein diets. Oy vey. The truth is, most doctors of scleroderma patients recommend that their patients follow a normal, well-balanced diet without the addition of herbs or minerals. If you're interested in taking supplements, make sure to check with your doctor first. It's usually not a good idea to eliminate entire food groups (unless it's due to allergy) or go on a cleansing diet; these practices have been known to accelerate the disease process. However, your doctor may prescribe a particular diet for you, to address specific problems you may have.

For example, if you have high cholesterol, he or she might prescribe a low-fat diet. If you have kidney problems, he or she may tell you to avoid a diet high in protein. But that's between you and your doctor. Other ailments react to known dietary factors. If you suffer from heartburn, try to stay away from chocolate, caffeine, peppermint, and ginger (although ginger is often used to prevent nausea). If you're taking steroids to treat your disease, make sure you decrease your sugar, fat, and salt intake: Not only do steroids increase your appetite, they are known to raise blood sugar, cholesterol, and triglyceride levels. And that makes you put on extra weight. Also, the American College of Rheumatology recommends that people using steroids get 1,500 milligrams of calcium per day. This can be from food or supplements, or a combination of the two.

One food you may want to add to your diet is salmon or other fatty fish. Fish oil contains anti-inflammatory properties that have been shown to help people with rheumatoid arthritis. If eating fish isn't your thing, you may want to try fish-oil capsules as a substitute. But, speaking from personal experience, if you have swallowing difficulties, beware of this capsule. The capsules are about the size of the Titanic and are quite difficult to swallow.

A word of caution

Once thought of as quackery, CAM is now a $30-billion-a-year industry. But before you abandon conventional medicine, make sure you know what you're getting into. The promise of a quick cure can be awfully appealing—especially when you're not feeling well. Whether you're considering acupuncture for dental pain, homeopathy for allergies, or herbal remedies for depression, make sure you weigh the risks and benefits. Let's face it, if you search the Internet, you can find cures for just about anything. So be a smart consumer, and beware of product hype. Just because a product says "natural" doesn't mean it's safe or free of toxicity. In fact, most of these "natural" therapies are largely untested. One of the biggest problems today with most dietary and herbal supplements is that they are unregulated. And choosing an untested alternative over an established treatment is just not smart medicine. When all is said and done, CAM can be a wonderful addition to your current treatment plan. If used correctly, it can make both the disease and the treatment more bearable. Just remember: Do your homework. There's no substitute for knowledge when you're dealing with your own health.

IN A SENTENCE:

> *Complementary and alternative medicine can be a wonderful addition to your current treatment plan; just make sure you're not doing yourself more harm than good.*

learning

Does Alternative Medicine Have a Place in Scleroderma?

THOSE WHO live with a chronic illness or chronic pain are some of the most likely patients to look beyond mainstream Western medicine. The truth is, most of us have probably tried alternative medicine without even knowing it. If you've tried massage, meditation, or supplements, consider it official: You've tried alternative medicine. I myself have tried at least half a dozen things, including biofeedback, massage, yoga, aromatherapy, herbs, visualization, reflexology, and more. Most of the patients I interviewed for this book have tried at least something; some even swear by the results. The physicians I surveyed, however, held decidedly mixed views on the use of CAM. Some were quite enthusiastic about its place in scleroderma treatment. Daniel Wallace, clinical professor of medicine at Cedars-Sinai Medical Center/UCLA, felt very strongly about the benefits of mind-body therapies for scleroderma, as well as for many other rheumatic diseases. Other physicians were a bit more skeptical. Their skepticism may be due to the lack of available scientific data, or from a lack of knowledge. Or quite possibly, it may be because many of their patients neglect to inform them about what type of treatments they're using. Whatever the reason, there's a right way and a wrong way to incorporate CAM into your current treatment plan. Let's start with the basics.

Patient guidelines for choosing wisely

If you're considering entering the world of alternative medicine, there are several things you need to be aware of before you take the plunge. When you're tired of feeling sick all the time, both physically and mentally, you're probably willing to try just about anything to feel better and regain some control. When you've reached the "I'll do *anything* to feel better" stage, keep in mind you're probably at your most vulnerable. And that's exactly when the marketers of these products want to find you. The products or services can sound so appealing: "MIRACLE CURE!" " GET ENERGIZED!" " NO MORE PAIN!" You want to believe it, and are ready to pay top dollar for it. Don't. You're a savvy consumer, remember? Take your time and do your homework. You're not shopping for a new TV. You're shopping for your health. Before you decide to purchase any new alternative product or service, consider the following guidelines:

1. **Don't assume all alternative remedies are harmless and will make you feel better.** This is the time to start gathering information about the product or service you're interested in. The Internet is a fabulous place to start, but beware: It can be one of the greatest sources of misinformation, too. Start by looking at the safest and most reputable sites. These include universities, major medical centers, national organizations, and government websites. You can also go to the library, ask your friends, or talk to your doctor. You can even ask your doctor if he or she knows any physicians who practice integrative medicine. Some of the larger universities and medical centers offer such programs. Just make sure your insurance company covers the cost before you make an appointment.

2. **Evaluate treatment providers.** I probably don't have to say this, but never choose an alternative treatment provider from the phone book. You're just asking for trouble if you do. Besides getting referrals from your friends or doctor, one of the best ways to find a reputable

provider is through the therapy's local or national association. For example, if you're looking for an acupuncturist, the major certifying board for acupuncturists is the National Certification Commission for Acupuncture and Oriental Medicine. It has certified thousands of practitioners who have met national professional standards in the field. If you're looking for a medical doctor who has completed an acupuncture training program, check with the American Academy of Medical Acupuncture for a provider in your area. And never hesitate to set up an informational interview before you make an appointment, to see if it's the right match for you.

3. ***Consider the cost.*** Many alternative treatments are not covered by insurance. Be sure to find out about the cost before you begin treatment.

4. ***Keep an open mind.*** You've chosen this path for a reason. Don't sabotage your own treatment. Learn to be open-minded and skeptical at the same time. And don't ever underestimate the placebo effect.

5. ***Know when to use complementary medicine versus conventional medicine.*** It's one thing to try alternative medicine; it's another to know when to use it. If you have a sudden, acute, or life-threatening problem, you need conventional medicine. You should call your doctor immediately. If you're trying to maintain your health or relieve symptoms, use CAM.

6. ***Don't expect a cure.*** Some alternative treatments may make you feel better or allow you to regain some control over your health care and life. But remember, these types of treatments won't cure your scleroderma. If there was a cure for the disease, you probably wouldn't need to be using these treatments in the first place. Make sure you have realistic goals for whatever treatment you choose.

7. ***Beware of snake oils.*** Trust your gut. Medical fraud is rampant in this industry. If it sounds too good to be true, it probably is.

Work closely with your doctor

As you learned in Month 2, the doctor-patient relationship is a delicate partnership based on trust and mutual respect. Up to this point, you've tried to be as honest as possible with each other and have been very satisfied with your relationship. Your doctor's opinion has been important to you and you want his or her approval. Now, though, you've reached the point where you'd like to try some alternative medicine and are hesitant to tell your doctor for fear he or she will disapprove of your new plans. It's true: Not all doctors approve of CAM. But don't assume yours is one of those doctors. The following tips may help you and your physician bridge the CAM gap; consider using them in the hopes of encouraging an open and honest dialogue about additional treatment options:

- Speak to your doctor before you begin any type of CAM. You might be pleasantly surprised by your doctor's positive reaction. In fact, he or she may even be able to recommend a good practitioner in your area of interest. And even if your doctor doesn't agree with you, he or she will appreciate your honesty.

- Open a dialogue with your physician about the treatment you're interested in. Ask your physician if he or she knows anything about it or can recommend someone who does. If your doctor doesn't know anything about it, offer information. From articles to supplement labels to studies from medical journals, share what you have learned. Not only will your physician realize how serious you are, he or she might actually learn something to share with other patients. It pays to do your homework—for both you and your doctor.

- Always be honest and up-front with your doctor. Never do something behind his or her back that may jeopardize your health. Make sure your doctor is aware of everything you are taking and doing— some treatments may have serious consequences you don't know about. Even if your doctor doesn't agree with your new treatment, he or she can at least provide you with sound medical advice. Many herbs interact very badly with prescription drugs, and some are downright dangerous. Even the benign over-the-counter medication you're taking may be doing you more harm than good. Let your doctor be the one to sort out what's safe and what's not. In the long run, you'll be glad you brought it up.

- If your doctor approves of the new treatment, ask for a prescription or a referral. The treatment may be covered by your health insurance if it's prescribed by your doctor. A friend of mine had six massages paid for by insurance. But remember, honesty is always the best policy. Make sure the treatment is medically necessary.

○ If your doctor flat-out refuses to talk about CAM and won't consider your needs, you have a few options:

1. If you've been satisfied with your overall medical treatment thus far, ask your doctor why he or she feels this way. He or she may have legitimate reasons. Perhaps he or she witnessed a negative experience or an unusually bad outcome. You may just have to agree to disagree and move forward with your treatment goals.

2. If your doctor won't budge from his or her opinions, it may be time to find a new doctor. Look for one who's more open-minded about CAM and who's willing to consider your need to look beyond conventional medicine.

○ Make sure you want to have this much responsibility for your own health care. If you're the type of patient who likes to be told what to do, CAM may not be right for you.

Scleroderma patients' experiences

Many scleroderma patients have gone beyond conventional medicine, from prayer to meditation to tai chi, to try to help themselves feel better. The following anecdotal experiences demonstrate that what is one person's savior can be another's nemesis. That said, here's what some scleroderma patients have tried. Do not try any of the following without speaking to your physician first.

○ *Joan* has tried acupuncture for various ailments, herbs for circulation, and pilates for stretching.

○ *Bonnie D.* takes tai chi, which helps her with movement and flexibility and helps her state of mind. She also takes an herb called milk thistle for her liver problems, although her gastroenterologist was not in favor of it. She says it has actually helped to lower her liver enzyme tests, which was her goal when she began to take it.

○ *Sheri* flew all the way to Jamaica to try lamb fetal cells. Not knowing what to expect, she could never figure out if the treatment was successful or not.

○ *Lydia* went to Andrew Weil's Program in Integrative Medicine at the University of Arizona in Tucson, Arizona. She has changed her diet to 90 percent raw foods and rarely eats any animal products. She also has added supplements to her diet. Besides doing light meditation, she's also found new breathing techniques that seem to be quite helpful for controlling her stress.

○ *Bev* does acupuncture for pain and has added fruit and vegetable supplements to her diet.

○ *Cookie* began taking ginkgo biloba and has had increased energy ever since.

○ *Christie* has been to homeopathic doctors and tried many different herbs . . . with no success. Although she loves meditation and is very spiritual, her philosophy is, "I have found that I'm my healthiest when I do what I want, when I want, and rid myself of energy-draining people and situations."

A few remedies that can't hurt you

Although this is not an endorsement for any particular treatment, the following therapies have been known to improve the conditions listed below:

○ **Anxiety and stress**—massage, biofeedback, meditation, yoga, visualization, and relaxation techniques (i.e., breathing excercises)

○ **Raynaud's phenomenom**—Biofeedback, acupuncture, fish oil

○ **Pain**—biofeedback, acupuncture

Are herbs right for you?

Herbs are used to treat all sorts of ailments, from depression to insomnia. But are they right for you? As you learned earlier in the chapter, some herbs can have a toxic effect when mixed with prescription or over-the-counter drugs. And not all manufactured herbs are created equal. Make sure to stick with familiar manufacturers and make sure the herb has an

HERB CHART

HERB	CLAIMED USES	POTENTIAL SIDE EFFECTS
Alfalfa	Antiarthritic	In larger quantities, can produce panctopenia (decreased white blood cell count, anemia); can reactivate lupus
Arnica	Analgesic, anti-inflammatory (external application)	May cause contact dermatitis; cannot be taken internally; causes toxic effects on the heart and increases blood pressure
Black cohosh	Antirheumatic, sore throat, uterine difficulties	Information on toxicity is lacking; can cause uterine bleeding
Burdock	Treatment of skin conditions	Side effects may result from addition with belladonna
Butcher's broom	Used to improve venous circulation, anti-inflammatory	Unknown; self-medication for circulatory problems is dangerous
Calamus	Digestive aid, antispasmodic for dyspepsia	Use only Type 1 (North American) calamus, which is free of carcinogenic iso a sarone (ingredients that may promote cancers)
Calendula (marigold)	Facilitate healing of wounds (lacerations)	Unknown
Capsicum	Counterirritant used to treat chronic pain (herpes zoster, facial neuralgia, or surgical trauma)	Use caution in application: avoid getting into eyes or other mucous membranes; remove from hands with vinegar
Catnip	Digestive, sleep aid	Unknown; does not mimic marijuana when smoked
Chamomiles, yarrow	Used to aid digestion, anti-inflammatory, antispasmodic, anti-infective	Infrequent contact dermatitis and hypersensitivity reactions in susceptible people
Chickweed	Treatment of skin disorders, stomach and bowel problems	Unknown
Comfrey	General healing agent, stomach ulcer treatment	Hepatotoxicity (liver); can lead to liver failure, especially when the root is eaten; also causes atropine poisoning due to mislabeling
Cranberry	Treatment of bladder infections	Increased calories if used in large doses (12-32 ounces per day) as a treatment rather than as a preventative (3 ounces per day)

HERB	CLAIMED USES	POTENTIAL SIDE EFFECTS
Dandelion	Digestive, laxative, diuretic	Free of toxicity except for contact dermatitis in people allergic to it
Devil's claw	Antirheumatic	None
Dong Quai	Antispasmodic	Large amounts may cause photosensitivity and lead to dermatitis, possible bleeding
Echinacea	Wound healing (external), immune stimulant (internal)	Don't use in autoimmune disease. Allergies are possible; be sure product is pure and not adulterated with prairie dock (can cause nausea, vomiting); may flare lupus
Evening primrose	Treatment of atopic eczema, breast tenderness, arthritis	No data; borage seed oil (20% as GLA) may be a substitute and does have toxic side effects (liver toxicity, carcinogen)
Fennel	Calms stomach, promotes burping	Do not use the volatile oil, which causes skin reactions, vomiting, seizures, and respiratory problems; no side effects with use of seeds
Fenugreek	Calms stomach	None
Garlic	Used to treat GI ailments, reduce blood pressure, prevent clots	Large doses are needed (uncooked, up to 4 grams of fresh garlic a day), which may result in GI upsets; can "thin" the blood (anticoagulant)
Gentian expectant	Appetite stimulant	May not be well tolerated by mothers or people with high blood pressure (possibly increasing pressure)
Ginkgo biloba	Helps dementia	Very well tolerated
Ginseng	Adaptogen, cure-all, antistress agent	Be sure the product is pure; some insomnia, diarrhea, and skin eruptions have been reported; possible immune stimulant (antagonized other medications)
Goldenseal	Digestive aid, treatment of genitourinary disorders	In huge doses, may cause uterine cramps
Honey	Used to treat sore throat; antiseptic, anti-infective, antiarthritic; sedative	Do not give to children under one year of age; may cause botulism in infants
Lovage	Diuretic; promotes burping	Some photosensitivity with volatile oil of lovage
L-tryptophan	Sleep aid, antidepressant	Be sure product is pure; contaminants may cause a serious blood disorder and a scleroderma-like illness

HERB	CLAIMED USES	POTENTIAL SIDE EFFECTS
Mistletoe	Stimulates smooth muscle (American); antispasmodic and calmative (European)	Berries are highly toxic and the leaves may also cause cell death; in animals, lowers blood pressure and weakens, constricts blood vessels
Nettle	Antiarthritic, antiasthmatic, diuretic	Skin irritation from active ingredients
New Zealand green-lipped mussel	Antiarthritic	No toxicity or side effects except in those allergic to seafood
Passionflower	Calmative, sedative	None
Peppermint	Calms stomach, promotes burping, antispasmodic	Do not give to infants and young children, who may choke on the menthol
Pokeroot	Antirheumatic, cure-all	Vomiting, blood cell abnormalities, hypotension, decreased respiration, gastritis
Rosemary	Antirheumatic, digestive stimulant	Large quantities of the volatile oil taken internally cause stomach, intestinal, and kidney irritation
Rue	Antispasmodic, calmative	Skin blisters and photosensitivity following contact; gastric upsets when taken internally; may be an effective antispasmodic but is too toxic to be used
Saint-John's-wort (Hypericum)	Antidepressant, anti-inflammatory, wound healing	Photosensitivity dermatitis in those who take the herb for extended periods; Prozac-like; increases serotonin
Sairei-to	Antiarthritic	Diarrhea, abdominal pain, rash
Sassafras	Antispasmodic, antirheumatic	Active ingredient is carcinogenic in rats and mice
Senna	Cathartic	Diarrhea, gastric and intestinal irritation with large and/or habitual doses
Tea tree oil	Antiseptic (external application only)	No side effects except skin irritation in sensitive individuals
Valerian (garden heliotrope)	Tranquilizer, calmative	None noted
Yucca	Antiarthritic	None noted

approved use. Also, be cautious of any herbs manufactured outside the United States European herbs are highly regulated, but you should watch out for toxic ingredients in any herbs coming from China or India. The preceding herb chart, originally compiled by Daniel Furst, M.D., and Elaine Furst, R.N., and subsequently adapted and reproduced by Daniel Wallace, M.D., gives you some basic information on herbs used to treat skin, gastrointestinal, and arthritic symptoms.

It's up to you to decide what treatments are best for you. And if you're like me, I'm sure you have plenty of well-intentioned friends recommending this type of treatment or that. One friend offered to fly me to Timbuktu to try out some type of chamber that sounded like a torture chamber, which had been touted to cure everything from toenail fungus to liver cancer. When I politely declined his offer and replied, "You first," he was so offended by my lack of consideration, he refused to talk to me for weeks. When the dust settled, I realized his reaction and anger came from his lack of control over my disease and a willingness to do everything possible to help me feel better. Friends and family may have good intentions, but ultimately it is up to you to decide what treatments you're willing to try and what feels the most comfortable to you.

IN A SENTENCE:

> *Complementary and alternative medicine can offer additional benefits to your treatment plan if used wisely and with caution.*

Shouldn't I Be Feeling Better by Now?

YOU'VE BEEN living with your disease for six months. It's been a struggle, but you've made it. You'd love to be able to pat yourself on the back at this point, but the reality is you're still feeling like you've been run over by a Mack truck. And all this time you thought the hard part was getting a diagnosis. As you're beginning to find out, sometimes living with the disease can be even harder. You might be at the stage where you're still going through some testing. Or perhaps some new symptoms have popped up and your doctors are still doing damage control. Whatever your situation may be, all you know is you're still feeling bad, period.

This is typical in scleroderma

Rest assured, you are not alone. For most patients, the first year is a never-ending, winding road full of surprises. Because no two patients are alike, it's hard to gauge exactly where you're supposed to be at any one point in your disease. This is completely normal. One way to put your mind at ease is to remind yourself that because there are so many different types of scleroderma, everyone's path is going to be a bit different. Before you start to wonder whether what you're experiencing is normal, call your doctor to find out. Don't get caught up in what another patient experienced when she was at this point in her disease. Remember what you learned in Week 4? In a disease like scleroderma, expect the unexpected.

What to be on the lookout for

At this point the one thing you *don't* want to do is ignore the way you're feeling. Make sure you let your doctor know exactly how you're feeling, as well as any new symptoms you may be experiencing. There just might be a legitimate reason for why you feel the way you do. Let's talk about a few different scenarios to consider:

- ○ **Your medications haven't kicked in yet.** Speaking from experience, I can attest that, although some medications kick in immediately, others take a while to work. If you've just started on a new medication and haven't felt its effects yet, be patient. Speak to your doctor or pharmacist about how long the medication typically takes to work. Whatever you do, don't stop taking the medication without checking with your doctor first. If you're past the point of when it should've started to take effect, it probably isn't the right medication for you.
- ○ **You're not on the right medications.** Finding the right treatment plan is like putting together a jigsaw puzzle. There's lots of trial and error before you get it right. It may be just one medication that needs changing, or, if you're on multiple medications, it could be the interactions among them that's making you feel bad. Or, perhaps the side effects of the medications are making you feel this way. I call this the chicken or the egg theory. Are you feeling this way because of the disease or are you feeling this way because of the treatment for the disease? Unfortunately, there's no easy way to find out.
- ○ **You're experiencing new symptoms.** Even though you went through a lot of testing in the first few months after your diagnosis, something new may have popped up since then. Make sure you talk to your doctor about it as soon as possible. Remember, early intervention and treatment is crucial in a disease like scleroderma.

O **You haven't quite figured out how to pace yourself.** Never underestimate the importance of pacing yourself. Running around like you used to pre-diagnosis is bound to wear you out. You must take into account that your life has changed. And that may mean rethinking your priorities.

O **You're dealing with a lot of stress in your life right now.** Stress and scleroderma don't go well together. Stress can exacerbate your symptoms and make you feel worse than you already do. The irony of coping with a chronic disease is that the disease itself is often the cause of your stress. You'll learn more about how stress can affect your disease in Month 11; try, as much as possible, to eliminate it. If you're going through a particularly stressful period right now (disease-related or not), remember to be kind to yourself.

O **It's the fatigue that's killing you.** Forget the disease, it's the fatigue you could do without. Although there's no magic bullet to cure your fatigue, learning to pace yourself will make a big difference in your life. Take naps. And eliminate any activities in your life that aren't absolutely necessary. You'll learn more about how to deal with fatigue in the Learning section of this chapter.

O **You're not taking any medications right now but you may need to.** Perhaps you and your physician decided to take a "wait and watch" approach. You both agreed to see how things progressed before you started on any medications. If this was your original approach and you are feeling progressively worse, it may be time for you and your physician to reevaluate your situation and determine whether it's time to begin treatment. Beginning a treatment plan can make a world of difference in how you're feeling.

How to cope

Whatever your situation may be, the bottom line is you just want to feel better than you do right now. Whether you're feeling bad from your medications, fatigue, or new symptoms, you need to work closely with your doctor to try to determine the cause. Now's not the time to roll over and accept how bad you feel. Remember, you're in charge of your disease. Don't let the disease be in charge of you. The following game plan will help you focus your efforts on helping yourself to feel better:

1. *Make a list of all the new symptoms you're experiencing.* And make sure it's thorough. A symptom you consider insignificant may be exactly what your doctor needs to know about. Even if you think it sounds stupid, write it down. Your doctor's not there to judge you. He or she wants to help you feel better. Just make sure you don't forget to bring your list with you when you visit your doctor.

2. *Make an appointment to see your physician.* Here's your chance to go over your list with your doctor. Remember to discuss the most important issues on your list before anything else. And don't let your doctor dismiss you without any concrete solutions, especially if you truly believe there is something new going on. Insist on additional testing if you think it will help, or ask to try a different medication than the one you're taking. This is your chance to take an active role in your health care.

3. *Try to reprioritize some of your responsibilities.* Often it's the little things in your life that can make you feel worse. You have a to-do list a mile long and just looking at it makes you feel tired. The best thing to do is redo your list and keep only the things that need to get done today on it; eliminate the rest. Do you really need to buy your uncle's birthday present today? Can the post office wait until tomorrow? If you can put off all the things on your list except the absolute necessities, by all means do so.

4. *Take care of your emotional health.* Trying to cope with the physical manifestations of the disease can take a toll on your emotions. And it's not healthy to keep your emotions bottled up. Sharing your emotions with someone you trust may be all it takes to lighten the load, both physically and emotionally. If you don't feel comfortable sharing your feelings with your family or friends, make an appointment to see a mental health professional, or join a support group. Support groups allow you to have your feelings validated by others who have been in your shoes.

When you were first diagnosed, six months ago, getting through the first month seemed like a worthy accomplishment. And now you've made it through six. You probably never thought that this was possible in the early days of your disease. And now you're here. Even though you may not be feeling as well as you would like, no one can predict what tomorrow will bring. If you keep reminding yourself to take it one day at a time, I think you'll have an easier time moving forward with your disease.

IN A SENTENCE:

> *You may still not be feeling well, even though you have been working closely with your doctor; this may be completely normal for the type of scleroderma you have.*

learning

Managing
Your Fatigue

DO YOU get a good night's sleep and still wake up feeling exhausted the next day? Does your body feel so tired that sometimes when you sit down, you feel you can't stand up again? Are you so tired on certain days that you feel like you can't move? Welcome to one of the most under-recognized symptoms of your disease: fatigue. And I'm not talking about the "I'm tired because I've stayed up too late" kind. I'm talking about the overwhelming, debilitating fatigue that can take over your daily life. You've probably spent the last six months worrying about the other, more tangible symptoms of scleroderma. You've been working closely with your doctor to try to get these other symptoms under control. The last thing on your mind was your fatigue. But its pervasive, unrelenting nature has kept reminding you of its presence until it can no longer be ignored. For some patients, the fatigue is merely bothersome. But for others, it can be life-changing. And although estimating the degree of fatigue can be subjective, most patients will agree that it's something that never completely goes away.

Cause and effect

Although fatigue is certainly a hallmark of the disease, other factors may be contributing to it. Let's explore some things that may be exacerbating this most unwelcome symptom:

1. **Inflammation**—The process of inflammation has been considered to be a major cause of fatigue. The process involves the infiltration of white blood cells into the tissues, and chemicals called **cytokines** are thought to be increased during the inflammatory process. Some doctors suspect that this increase in cytokines is largely responsible for disease-related fatigue. The bottom line: You must work closely with your doctor to make sure your disease is being adequately controlled.

2. **Anemia**—This is a condition in which the blood is low in red cells and/or hemoglobin, resulting in excessive fatigue and weakness. Causes can include anything from certain medications to the disease itself. If your physician suspects that you are anemic, a simple blood test can confirm the diagnosis. Once the diagnosis is established, you must work with your physician to determine the cause.

3. **Depression**—It's quite normal to feel depressed when dealing with a chronic disease. Don't forget that fatigue is one of the major symptoms of depression: And vice versa: Depression may manifest itself as fatigue.

4. **Stress**—Whether it's ongoing or situational, stress can be exhausting. Look for ways to better deal with your stress, as it can also exacerbate your symptoms.

5. **Pain**—Any type of pain can be draining. It can zap your energy and leave you feeling listless and lethargic. Make sure your pain is being adequately controlled at all times. If your current medication isn't working, don't be a hero. There's no need to suffer in silence. Keep working with your physician until you find the medication that works for you.

6. **Other medical conditions**—Thyroid conditions often accompany autoimmune diseases. Make sure your physician rules out any underlying thyroid problems as a cause of your fatigue. Once diagnosed, thyroid problems can be easily treated with medication.

7. **Medication side effects**—Often overlooked is the fact that many medications can cause incredible fatigue—especially if you're on more than one. Ask your doctor for an alternate choice and keep trying until you find the right one or the right mix that doesn't make you feel so weary.

How to cope

Although targeting the cause of your fatigue is the best way to combat it, there are other things you can do in your daily life to help you cope. Let's talk about what you can do to help stop fatigue from completely taking over your day-to-day life.

○ *Pace yourself.* Just because your to-do list is a mile long doesn't mean you have to get it all done today. If something can wait until another day, then by all means postpone it. Especially if you're having a low-energy day. Don't waste your good energy on unnecessary tasks. If you keep pushing yourself too hard today, you'll end up feeling just as bad tomorrow, too.

○ *Make sure you're getting enough sleep.* If you're not getting enough sleep at night, you're going to feel tired the next day, period. If insomnia is an issue for you, try the following suggestions:

- Avoid caffeine and alcohol too close to bedtime.
- Take a warm bath.
- Drink some warm milk.
- Try getting some exercise during the day.
- Talk to your doctor about medications to help you sleep.

○ *Delegate chores to other family members.* Don't have enough energy to do the laundry? Ask for help. Whether from a spouse, child, friend, or house cleaner, make sure you get the help you need around the house. And when all else fails, make sure you buy some extra underwear next time you're at the store.

○ *Rest when you need to.* When you feel yourself getting tired, make sure you stop to take a rest. Even if that means a short nap.

Recharging your batteries may be all you need to feel refreshed enough to make it through the rest of your day.

o *Get some exercise.* Exercising may be harder for some than for others, but remember: Increasing your activity level can boost your energy level. Just make sure you don't get caught in the vicious cycle of letting your body get out of shape, which causes you to be more fatigued, thus making it even more difficult for you to become physically active.

o *Try to reduce the stress in your life.* Although easier said than done, reducing the amount of stress in your life will increase your energy level. And not just physically. Stress can also cause mental and emotional fatigue. The more you can reduce the stress in your daily life, the better you'll feel, physically and mentally.

o *Eat a well-balanced diet.* Sometimes when you're feeling ill, the last thing you want to do is eat—especially if you're experiencing any scleroderma-related GI problems. But maintaining your energy requires a nutritious diet. Good nutrition must be a top priority for your overall health and well-being.

Learning to accept the fatigue

Some people may try every trick in the book to combat their fatigue, to no avail. And some may feel frustrated that they don't have the same amount of energy they had before the onset of their disease. This is a normal reaction. But instead of using your limited amount of energy on a negative emotion like anger, do something nice for yourself and try to accept your new life. Take a warm bath. Get a massage. Go see a movie. Relax with a good book. If you've made sure you've done everything you can to find the cause of your fatigue, there's no sense in beating yourself up over what you can't control.

IN A SENTENCE:

> *Fatigue is a common symptom in scleroderma; learning to accept and manage it may take some time.*

HALF-YEAR MILESTONE

Now that you are halfway through your first year with scleroderma, you have

○ DISCOVERED THE IMPORTANCE OF THE DOCTOR-PATIENT RELATIONSHIP AND LEARNED ABOUT YOUR RIGHTS AS A PATIENT;

○ LEARNED ALL ABOUT THE CLINICAL TRIAL PROCESS AND BEGUN TO CONSIDER WHETHER ONE MIGHT BE RIGHT FOR YOU;

○ REALIZED THAT YOU HAVE RIGHTS AS AN EMPLOYEE AND LEARNED WHAT TO EXPECT FROM THE SOCIAL SECURITY DISABILITY PROCESS; AND

○ BECOME AWARE OF THE WORLD OF COMPLEMENTARY AND ALTERNATIVE MEDICINE.

Disease Progression

HAVING A chronic disease brings up all sorts of fears, both rational and irrational. One of the worst fears for people with a chronic disease is fear of the unknown. And the biggest unknown is disease progression. Your doctor may be able to tell you the "typical" course for your particular type of scleroderma, but remember it is just that: typical. Scleroderma is a disease filled with variables. Adding to its variability is scleroderma's mysteriousness. Take two people with the same set of symptoms at diagnosis. If both patients were followed for the next twelve months, it's more likely than not that they would be at different points in their disease by the end of those twelve months, each having experienced unique symptoms. The unpredictability of it all is hard enough. The reality can be downright scary.

What you have control over

Getting a disease like scleroderma can be hardest on those who consider themselves to be control freaks. It's almost like taking a crash course in how to let go—only not by choice. But although you don't have control over the course of your disease or its manifestations, you actually have much more control in your life than you think you have. Consider the following:

○ **You have control over how well you take care of yourself.** Are you living the healthiest way you know how? Are you getting enough exercise? Plenty of rest? Eating a well-balanced diet? If you answered yes to these questions, pat yourself on the back. You're doing all that you possibly can to live a healthy lifestyle. That will only help you cope with your disease in the long run. But if you answered no to the above questions and your lifestyle seems a bit untidy at the moment, you may need to rethink your priorities. Perhaps the occasional foray into drugs, alcohol, or cigarettes may be the only way you know how to cope. But if that occasional foray turns into something more, you're doing both yourself and your disease a disservice. Try to get the help you need to learn better coping skills. It's essential to your long-term health and well-being.

○ **You have control over your mental outlook.** This is where the old "Do you see the glass as half-full or half-empty?" comes into play. One of the most important things in dealing with a chronic disease is attitude. It's okay to feel anger and sadness about your diagnosis, but try your best to move through it. And continue to have hope. Although it's natural for people with an incurable disease to hope for a cure, try breaking it down into smaller increments: Hope to control your pain or alleviate it completely. Hope to make it through your day with less fatigue. Hope for fewer disease exacerbations. And hope for both physical and mental healing along the way.

○ **You have control over the amount of activities you do in your life.** One of the most important things you can do for yourself is learn to pace yourself. That may mean cutting out an activity or two—so be it. It's more important to feel well rested and to enjoy the activities you can do, rather than feel like you're stretched too thin and are exhausted all the time.

○ **You have control over what you eat.** I know, I know, easier said than done. Especially coming from a self confessed ex-junk food junkie. But getting scleroderma made me realize the importance of eating healthier. And although chocolate is still a staple in my diet

(I consider it one of my four major food groups), at least fruits and vegetables are, too. One thing to watch out for is medications that can cause weight gain. Prednisone (steroids), in particular, is one of the worst culprits in causing medication-related weight gain. If you have to take this drug at any point in your disease, it's critical to limit your salt and fat intake. Very few escape the prednisone weight gain. Except me. You may hate me for telling you this, but I actually lost weight while taking steroids. And my appetite. I wouldn't recommend this type of weight loss strategy to anyone. Weight loss rarely happens, and prednisone has lots of other nasty side effects *besides* probable weight gain. Nevertheless, it can be a life-saving drug, well worth the weight gain.

○ **You have control over how you spend your time.** Learning to pace yourself is crucial; so is deciding how you choose to spend your time. If taking that new class you love leaves you feeling exhausted and cranky or is cutting into your family time, you need to rethink your priorities. Try postponing a planned activity for a time when you're feeling better or have less going on in your life. While you may feel sad about not being able to participate in something you'd like to be doing right now, it's not worth doing if it only makes you feel worse. Promise yourself you'll reevaluate the situation in another six months. You'll be glad you did.

○ **You have control over how you choose to manage your disease.** Denial was an acceptable coping skill in the beginning of your journey; at this point in your disease, it's not. Accepting your disease and its limitations is the healthiest way to move forward. If you're having a hard time reaching that point, it's time to get some help. Speak to your physician, talk to a therapist, join a support group, or do whatever you have to to help yourself manage your disease. The sooner the better.

○ **You have control over early intervention and treatment of your disease.** It may not seem like it, but you do have more control than you realize over how your disease is treated. After all, it's your body. The best strategy is almost always early intervention, although you may not agree. If you choose to take the wait and watch approach against your doctor's recommendation, you're just asking for trouble. Ask yourself why you've chosen this approach. Are you frightened of the medications? Don't like taking pills every day? Whatever the reason, try to figure out what it is and then speak honestly with your doctor about it. The best solution is to try to work out a compromise that won't jeopardize your health in the meantime. If you don't like a particular medication your doctor has recommended, ask to try a different one. You can usually find a solution to these types of problems.

What you don't have control over

While there are many things you can control, there are just as many that you can't. That's the harsh reality of having a chronic disease. Let's take a look at the things you don't have control over:

○ You don't have control over your disease manifestations.
○ You don't have control over the side effects of your medications.
○ You don't have control over the type of scleroderma you get.
○ You don't have control over the physical changes the disease may cause.
○ You don't have control over the course your disease may take.

You may still be grappling with the lack of control you have in these areas. If so, try looking at it from a different angle. That's what I did. Instead of feeling bad about the things I couldn't control, I started focusing on the things that I could control. Not only did it relieve the burden of feeling that I had to be in control all the time—it actually made me realize that it was okay not to be in control.

The reality of disease progression

Typically (there's that word again), those who have localized scleroderma don't have the same worries as those who have the systemic form. Localized scleroderma usually runs a more predictable course. The skin thickening tends to reach its maximum point in the first two to five years and then stabilize. Systemic scleroderma, on the other hand, is highly unpredictable, even among individuals with the same type. It is impossible to accurately predict who will experience which disease manifestation. That's why it's up to you to remain vigilant about your disease. Stay informed. Keep on top of the latest treatments. Learn about new research. Speak to other patients about their experiences. Because just when you think you can begin to relax a little, a new symptom will appear. And knowing how to deal with it can make all the difference in the progression of your disease.

IN A SENTENCE:

> *Although disease progression is unpredictable, you must learn what you can control and what you can't.*

learning

What Do These New Symptoms Mean?

AFTER A while, you develop a hypersensitivity to just about anything and everything that's happening to your body. Whenever a new symptom appears, you continually ask yourself, "Should I call the doctor *now* or should I wait a few days to see if it gets better?" Because it's so difficult to know what's normal and what's not for your particular disease type, you begin to worry about every little thing that pops up. This is completely normal. I still do this even after four years of living with the disease. The difference is, I've learned over the years that it's better to be safe than sorry. Before my diagnosis, I hardly ever called the doctor when I was sick. And if I did, I waited until I could hardly function before I made the call. One time I thought I had the flu but actually had pneumonia. I kept thinking I'd get better on my own and never called the doctor. I continued to get progressively worse and by the time I went to see my doctor, I could hardly breathe. After a simple chest X-ray, I was diagnosed with pneumonia and put on bed rest for the next couple of weeks. My internist at the time lectured me on the value of calling sooner, and how I could've ended up in the hospital if I had waited any longer. Ironically, this was the same doctor who told me nothing was wrong when I went to see him as soon as my first symptoms of scleroderma began. Regardless of the circumstances, I did learn the importance of calling the doctor before my symptoms get out of hand. This policy holds true for any new symptoms you may be experiencing. Early intervention is key in a disease like scleroderma. Don't waste time trying to self-diagnose. See your doctor promptly when something new arises.

It's better to be safe than sorry

As I've mentioned, no two people with scleroderma are affected in the same way. This makes it all the harder to determine what's normal and what's not, at this stage for your particular disease type. Most other diseases have a more predictable course than scleroderma. "Better safe than sorry'" should become your new motto. That doesn't mean deluging your physician with phone calls and daily visits that will only irritate and alienate him or her. But it does mean you should be an observant patient and get to know what's normal and what's not for your own body.

Do new symptoms mean my disease is getting worse?

New symptoms can be scary, no matter when they occur. But they can often be the scariest during your first year of scleroderma. You have no idea what to expect from your disease and it's easy to worry about every new thing. During my first year with scleroderma, I was constantly short of breath. I went from doctor to doctor to try to determine what was causing it. Although some of the doctors knew a little bit about scleroderma, most didn't know a thing. It took a very savvy pulmonologist, as well as a lung biopsy, to diagnosis interstitial lung disease. Now when I get short of breath, at least I know what's causing it and I'm not nearly as concerned as I was during my first year with the disease. It's important to remember the motto you learned earlier: better safe than sorry. Even if your new symptom turns out to be nothing, at least you'll have peace of mind.

When something new comes up, you may be especially concerned about whether your disease is getting worse. Although only your doctor can tell you for sure, one thing to keep in mind is that some connective-tissue diseases take time to evolve—especially if you have an overlap syndrome. Frustrating as this may feel, it's not uncommon to experience new symptoms as your particular type of disease is evolving. Make sure to keep your doctor informed so he or she can determine if any treatment is necessary.

Red Alert Symptoms

ALTHOUGH some new symptoms can be relatively harmless, others can be quite serious. If you're experiencing any of the following symptoms, make sure to call your doctor right away:

○ breathing difficulties
○ shortness of breath
○ chest pains
○ swollen ankles
○ feeling faint
○ ongoing diarrhea
○ persistent headache, nausea, and vomiting
○ swallowing difficulties
○ persistent cough
○ numbness
○ alternating diarrhea and constipation
○ persistent pain
○ other symptoms that are out of the ordinary for you

If you're experiencing any of the above symptoms, don't freak out. Only your doctor can determine if something more serious is going on. Your new symptom may even be completely unrelated to scleroderma. It's easy to blame just about every new ailment on scleroderma. I know, because I do this too. But whether or not your new symptom is related to your disease, you've done the right thing in getting it checked out. And you know what I'm going to say next: It's better to be safe than sorry (has it sunk in yet?).

Try to stay calm

Some new symptoms may be cause for alarm, but most aren't. If anything, your new symptom will wreak more havoc on your emotional state than on your body. This is normal. Having an unpredictable disease like scleroderma makes you feel as though your emotions are on high alert all the time. But you won't always feel this way. As time goes by and you get to know your particular disease a little better, new symptoms won't feel as threatening to you. This was the case with my shortness of breath. Of course, you still must remain vigilant and work to always stay on top of your disease. Scleroderma tends to surprise you when you least expect it. Remain calm and try your hardest to be ready for whatever new symptom may come your way.

IN A SENTENCE:

> *Make sure you call your doctor when any new symptoms arise,*
> *especially during your first year with scleroderma, when new*
> *symptoms are often the scariest.*

MONTH **8**

living

Taking Stock

YOU'VE MADE it through eight months of living with scleroderma. Give yourself a pat on the back for a job well done. But though you may be on the verge of disease burnout, you can't stop yet. This is a good time to sit down and evaluate where you are. Take a serious look at any changes you may need to make in your medical regime. You need to figure out what's working for you and what's not, from your doctors to your diet to your medications. But that's not all. You need to consider other disease-related things in your life, such as your health insurance and your pharmacist. And don't forget your emotional health, either. Even the most resilient patients need an attitude adjustment now and then. Whatever it is in your medical world that needs changing, now's a good time to clean house.

Start with your medical team

By now, you should have a good idea about how your medical team is working out. If you're dealing with a single physician, you should have a good idea of whether you and your doctor are a good match. As patients, we all need to have our own particular needs met. If yours aren't being met, it's time to make a change. To help you evaluate your doctor's performance, ask your-self the following questions:

O Is your doctor a good listener?
O Does he or she answer all your questions without making you feel bad for asking them?
O Are you happy with the way your disease is being managed?
O Are you comfortable with your doctor's knowledge of scleroderma?
O Are you satisfied with your treatments?
O Is your doctor responsive to your phone calls?
O Is your doctor willing to go the extra mile for you (like writing a let-ter to your insurance company or your employer)?
O Do you trust your physician(s)?
O Do the members of your medical team communicate with each other?

Every patient values some things more highly than others; you need to figure out what's most important to you. When I went through this process, one of the most important issues to me was my doctors' knowl-edge of the disease. I had the pleasure of meeting some very nice, trust-worthy, intelligent physicians who knew next to nothing about scleroderma. And that became my primary reason for changing doctors. Other patients may have other criteria—like long waits in the waiting room, or unreturned phone calls. Some patients may be quick to "fire" their physicians for just about anything; make sure you're not just trading in one bothersome problem for another. Also, keep in mind that some issues may be beyond your physician's control. If your only beef with your current doctor is that you're spending too much time in the waiting room, you had better make sure you're not going to have a similar problem with the next doctor you choose.

Consider the other areas of your medical world

One of the most important issues you need to address right now is whether your current medications are doing the trick. Because this topic is so important, the entire Learning section of this chapter is devoted to just that question. In the meantime, you need to think about other areas in your medical world that may need changing—like your pharmacy. Consider the following:

○ Does your pharmacist have time to answer your questions?
○ Is your phamacist able to tell you about the interactions among the different meds you're on?
○ Can the pharmacy fill your prescriptions in a timely manner?
○ Is the pharmacist helpful when unexpected insurance issues arise?
○ Does the pharmacy have a delivery service?
○ Does the pharmacy have convenient hours?
○ Is the pharmacy open 24 hours?
○ Are the lines tolerable?

If you answered yes to the above questions, you've chosen the right pharmacy. But if you find yourself spending far too long waiting in line at your pharmacy, only to be given the wrong prescription, or find the sheer stupidity of the staff makes you feel like you're in an episode of *Candid Camera*, then it's time to make a change. I guarantee it will make your life a whole lot easier—especially if you're taking multiple medications (which often means multiple trips to the pharmacy).

Other areas in your medical world to consider are things like your health insurance and your choice of hospitals. Or perhaps now's the time to file for disability. Or make a job change. Consider as well things like whether you need to become a more compliant patient or whether to change (or start!) your exercise program. Maybe you need to see a nutritionist. Or a therapist. Any positive changes you make now will only ensure your greater well-being in the future.

Attitude adjustment

Even the most optimistic among us can become jaded and cynical when confronted with the daily travails of scleroderma. This is normal. If you've been dealing relatively well up until this point but now find yourself feeling this way, don't despair. Allow yourself time to feel the funk and remind yourself it's only temporary. Perhaps after making a few changes like the ones mentioned above, you'll feel like your old self again. But if you find the feeling dragging on longer than you'd like it to, you may want to get some help. See a therapist. Join a support group. Talk it out with a trusted confidant. Discuss it with your physician. There's lots of help available. Make sure to get the help you need when you need it.

On the other hand, if you've been feeling in a funk ever since you received your diagnosis, it's definitely time for an attitude adjustment. Just as you need to reevaluate what's working and what's not in your medical world, so too do you need to examine your own attitude. Of course you can't be positive about everything all the time, but you can't be negative all the time, either. Do whatever you have to do to try and change your attitude. A good attitude goes a long way in dealing with a chronic disease and helps you get through the day-to-day stuff a lot more easily.

Time for a breather

This is also a good time to take a time-out. Dealing with the ins and outs of a chronic disease is stressful and exhausting. Now that you've decided what positive changes you need to make in your medical world, you can begin afresh. In the meantime, you need to relax. And that means both physically *and* mentally. If you can, try not to think about your disease for one whole day. Take the day off from work. Go out to dinner instead of cooking. Go to the beach. Go see a movie. Visit a museum. Stay in your pj's and read a book. Get a babysitter for the kids and go shopping. Meet your friends for tea. Play golf. Do whatever it is that will revive and refresh you. But whatever you decide to do, remember to make your special time only about you: Don't run errands. Don't pay the bills. Don't do yardwork. Don't clean your house. Don't get the car fixed. And by all means, don't make any doctor's appointments. You'll be better able to make these positive changes when you feel like you've had a little break. It's okay not to think about your disease for one day. Because you have the rest of your life to think about it when you need to.

IN A SENTENCE:

> It's often beneficial to review your medical situation at this point and make the necessary changes you need to successfully move forward.

learning

Are These Meds Really Helping Me?

AS YOU continue to take stock over the course of this month, one of the most important questions you need to ask yourself is whether your current medications are doing the trick. Most of us just expect the pills we're prescribed will do what they're supposed to do: make us better. We give little thought to the possibility that the pills may not be working. And very few of us consider whether our medications are causing us more harm than good. Now's the time to consider those possibilities. Whether you're taking one pill a day or twenty, here are some questions to ask yourself:

- ○ Is the medication doing what it was prescribed to do?
- ○ If the medication was prescribed for pain, is your level of pain noticeably reduced?
- ○ If you're taking more than one medication, are you experiencing any unpleasant interactions from them?
- ○ Are the side effects tolerable?
- ○ Do you feel better or worse while taking the medication?

Your answers to these questions will help you determine if it's time to make a change. Then you need to work closely with your doctor to decide if your medications need just a little tweaking or a major overhaul.

All medications are not created equal

After careful evaluation of your medications, you've realized they're not doing what they should be doing. What's the next step? First, consider precisely what it is that's not working and what it is you're trying to treat. Are you trying to treat a symptom or the overall disease? If you're trying to treat a particular symptom, you may just want to switch to a different drug in the same class. For example, say you were taking Vioxx, an anti-inflammatory drug (NSAID) known as a COX-2 inhibitor, for arthritic pain. But it's not working for you: you still have pain. Your doctor may then recommend Celebrex, a different COX-2 inhibitor, to see if it works any better. If that doesn't work, your doctor may try another type of anti-inflammatory drug that's *not* a COX-2 inhibitor like Relafen or Naprosyn. And one of those will finally do the trick for you. It's only through trial and error that you're able to figure out which medications are going to work best for you. Although it may feel discouraging to continually switch medications, it is completely normal. And what works for one patient may not work for another. I went through three different NSAIDs before I found one that worked. But once I did, I was able to stay on it for years.

The other scenario you may be confronted with is finding a drug to treat your overall disease. In certain situations, the only way to control disease activity is to control the underlying disease. If you find yourself in this situation, you need to talk to your doctor about using the "big guns": the disease-modifying drugs. For a review of those drugs, please see the Learning section in Week 3.

What your doctor doesn't tell you

In Day 6, you learned the value of educating yourself on all aspects of your disease—including your medications. This is crucial. Keep in mind that your doctor's office is something like school. When you were in school, not everything you learned was from your teacher. The same thing goes here: Not everything you learn about your disease is going to come from your doctor. Whenever

I'm prescribed a new medication (often, even before it's prescribed), the first thing I do is research it. I try to find out the following information:

1. What class of drug it is
2. How the drug works
3. What it's prescribed for
4. Dosing information
5. Side effects
6. Interactions with other drugs

After I've done my own research, I speak to my pharmacist. You're probably asking yourself if all that is really necessary. You bet it is. I can't count the number of times I've learned something on my own about a medication that I was never told about—and not just superfluous facts. I'm talking critical information about dosing, or drug interactions. Facts that can make a big difference in your life. Now the truth is, your doctor doesn't have to know every nuance of every drug he or she prescribes. But your doctor should at least know the answers to the questions listed above. Knowing any less is inexcusable. You're paying your doctor for his or her expertise. And it's not unreasonable to expect your doctor to find out the answers if he or she doesn't already know them. Unfortunately, the reality of today's world is, most doctors are overworked. No doubt your doctor is, too. Between seeing patients, doing paperwork, and managing the office, there's little time for doctors to do their "homework." Sure, you'll receive the basic care. But having a chronic disease requires more than just the basics. And you deserve the best care. Make sure you're receiving the most up-to-date drug information from your doctor, so that you're able to make the right decisions about which medications are best for you.

Your goals versus your doctor's goals

Ever stop to wonder, when you're given a prescription, whether you and your doctor have the same goal in mind? If you're like most patients, probably not. Usually your doctor's goal is pretty cut-and-dried. It works like this: You have a problem, your doctor tries to solve your problem, and you're most likely given a pill as the solution. For the short term, that's fine. Your doctor's goal was to solve your problem and that's precisely what he did. Job accomplished.

Now let's talk about your goals. Obviously, the first thing you want is a solution to whatever problem you may be having. And if the medication you're given helps your ailment, you too are probably satisfied for the short term. But have you ever thought about the long-term effects of your medications? If not, you should. Scleroderma patients are often put on medications indefinitely. And while your doctor may feel he or she has done his or her job by solving your problem of today, he or she may have given little thought to the problems your medications may cause in the future. Your goal is to think long-term. You're the one who has to deal with the long-term effects of your meds, not your doctor. Don't be afraid to bring this up with your doctor. If you're concerned about the long-term damage caused by a particular medication, your doctor may need to think more creatively about how and what he or she is prescribing for you.

Getting the right mix of meds is often like solving a puzzle

There's nothing more frustrating than finding the right medication to solve one problem only to have it cause another problem someplace else. This is a very common pattern. In some cases, the problems caused are merely nuisances, like finally finding a terrific drug to treat your **reflux**, only to have it cause occasional diarrhea. Other problems can be much more severe—like having to prioritize organs, for example. In my ongoing battle to keep my lungs stabilized, I was put on a wonderful drug that finally seemed to be doing the trick. Only now, that same wonderful drug is wreaking havoc on my kidneys. And although I often joke with my doctors about which is the more important organ to preserve, my lungs or my kidneys, the truth is, this wonder drug may be my only option; it is the only medication in its class. Sometimes these types of problems just aren't solvable. And only you can decide what you can live with. In most situations, though, your doctor will probably be able to come up with all sorts of options for you to choose from. But in the end, you're the one who is going to decide how to solve the puzzle.

IN A SENTENCE:

> *You must work closely with your physician to come up with the right mix of medications to work for both the short term and the long term.*

MONTH**9**

living

Getting Intimate

A CHRONIC disease like scleroderma can have a significant impact on your sex life—and not just physically. The psychological effects of having a chronic disease can wreak havoc on your self-esteem, and that also can be devastating to your sex life. Believe it or not, it *is* possible to have both scleroderma and a healthy sex life. All it takes is a little imagination, patience, communication, and desire. Although there are many causes for changes in your sex life or a loss of libido, most patients appreciate the opportunity to talk openly and honestly about how their sex life is affected by scleroderma. Hopefully, this chapter will help you to do just that.

Scleroderma-related physical problems can impact your sex life

Most patients tend to notice the physical changes of their disease first, but few realize the impact it can have on their sexuality. For some, these changes may not alter their sex life at all. For others, though, these changes can be a constant source of worry and shame. Consider the many physical problems that can occur in both sexes:

○ *Fatigue*—For many patients, just getting through the day is hard enough, much less having any extra energy left over for sex. While there's no "one size fits all" solution, using your time creatively may help to alleviate this problem. Whether it's learning to plan ahead for sex, making sure you're well rested beforehand, or having sex earlier in the day, try to work out a solution that both you and your partner can agree on. Although some of the spontaneity may get thrown out the window, at least you have anticipation to replace it with.

○ *Pain*—If pain is becoming a problem, try taking a warm bath beforehand. Or better yet, try taking a bath with your partner: The warm water will help your pain, and you'll both feel more relaxed. It's also a wonderful way to explore gentler ways of being intimate with one another. You may also want to try taking a pain reliever. Just make sure it's one your doctor has approved.

○ *Weight gain*—Whether it's caused by medications, inability to exercise, depression, or just plain old bad nutrition, weight gain will most certainly change the way you feel about yourself. You may not feel as attractive, or that your partner feels you're attractive. Such feeling can bring your sex life to a screeching halt. Remember, you're still the same person on the inside. So what if you look a bit different on the outside? This is the time for open and honest communication with your partner.

○ *Medications*—Many medications not only leave you feeling fatigued, but also can cause a loss of libido or leave you feeling mentally confused. And that can dampen even the best of sex lives. Work with your doctor in experimenting with other medications that may not have as many side effects. While you may get lucky and find the perfect mix of meds that make you feel just right for the moment, remember you may be trading one side effect for another. You may get your libido back—but now you may get acne. Or diarrhea. Or hot flashes. And just because you don't feel or see the side effect doesn't mean it's not happening. For instance, maybe your new medication doesn't make you feel groggy after you take it, but it causes bone loss in the long term. Don't fret. Try to compromise with yourself and don't expect perfection. Your goal here is to have a little fun. Don't make it harder on yourself than you have to. Or your partner, either, for that matter.

○ **Joint problems**—Joint problems can lead to decreased mobility, but a little experimenting usually solves the problem. Try using extra pillows or experimenting with different positions. You can even try some range-of-motion exercises before becoming intimate. And when all else fails, remember, there's more than one way to be intimate.

○ **Hand contractures**—This is a very common problem in scleroderma but one that is rarely addressed in literature. If your hands are affected by the disease in this way, now's the time to think creatively. Try thinking of alternative ways to touch each other, like using the back of your hands, or using your thumbs. Or try using any of the sexual aids that appeal to your fertile imaginations. Here's where brainstorming can be a lot of fun. Just make sure you and your partner are both on the same page about what your ultimate goals are.

○ **Reflux**—While few people are willing to admit it, gastrointestinal disturbances can ruin the mood faster than just about anything else. If you have a bad problem with reflux, try to make sure you watch your diet before you engage in any intimate activities. This means no spicy foods, caffeine, or alcohol. It may take some planning on your part, but it will be well worth it in the end.

○ **Decreased oral aperture (small mouth)**—If scleroderma has caused your mouth to shrink, both kissing and oral sex can become difficult. Work with a physical therapist to learn some exercises that help stretch your mouth and retain movement. If this isn't an option for you, keep in mind there are many different ways to express affection.

○ **Shortness of breath**—If this is a problem for you due to lung involvement or other scleroderma-related complications, the best advice is to take things very slowly and make sure you don't get too winded. Talk to your partner ahead of time about taking breaks if things get too hot and heavy for you. Also, don't let your fear of getting too out of breath stop you from enjoying yourself. With open communication and a sense of humor, you and your partner should be able to work out a solution that satisfies you both.

In women only:

○ **Vaginal dryness**—This can occur not only from Sjögren's phenomenon, but also from menopause—and even some medications. Before you can fix the situation, you must determine the cause. If it's caused by Sjögren's, try a water-based lubricant. If the cause is menopause, estrogen replacement hormones, available in pill form or vaginal cream, can be helpful.

In men only:

○ **Impotence**—While loss of libido is the more common cause of impotence in the general population, erectile dysfunction caused by neurological abnormalities or vascular problems is more likely the cause among scleroderma patients. Side effects from medications can also be the cause of erection problems. You and your partner must work closely with your doctor not only in determining the cause but in discussing treatment options, as well. This may also necessitate a work-up by a urologist.

Psychological and emotional problems can occur

Just as the physical changes from scleroderma can alter your sex life, so can the psychological and emotional difficulties of having a chronic disease. Consider the following:

○ **Depression**—It's a well-known fact that depression can cause a loss of libido. If depression is inhibiting your sex life, make sure you're being honest with your partner about your depression. Let your partner know that this is most likely the cause for your loss of libido. Also keep in mind that being intimate is about more than just being physical. If you find your depression goes on too long or is ruining your relationship, get some help. Talk to your physician about antidepressant medication and/or therapy. If you choose to take medication for your depression, remember this: Some antidepressants can also cause a loss of libido—so you may have to try several before finding the right one for you.

○ *Fear and anxiety*—You may be concerned that sex won't be as enjoyable as it was before the onset of your disease, or that it may be painful. And now you begin to shy away from it. This is a very normal reaction. Sometimes, the best way to get over our fears is to do the very thing that we're fearful of. Start slowly and do only what you're comfortable doing. And make sure your partner is aware of your feelings. Over time, your fears will slowly dissipate and you'll begin to enjoy yourself once again.

○ *Body-image dissatisfaction*—Whether it's caused by skin changes, lack of mobility, steroid-induced weight gain, or overall appearance changes, you may be feeling very unattractive. And then your self-image begins to go down the toilet. I'll remind you of a little saying all of our mothers used to tell us: "Beauty comes from within." If you keep repeating it, you may even start believing it. And hopefully, sooner rather than later.

○ *Feeling unworthy*—Because you're feeling so unattractive right now, you wonder how your partner could possibly find you attractive anymore. And this leaves you feeling angry and depressed. Don't let your emotions create this vicious circle. It will only make the situation worse and leave you feeling more isolated. You are worthy. And you are still attractive. Share your feelings with your partner and I'm sure you'll hear the same thing. Your feelings for yourself may have changed, but your partner's feelings for you haven't. Take some joy in that and go get busy.

You and your partner must work together

Don't assume the problem is only yours, either. Anything that happens to you affects your relationship with your partner. If your partner is concerned about your fatigue, pain, discomfort, or emotional distress, he/she may be hesitant to become intimate with you. This is not your fault. It was not your choice to get scleroderma. And having scleroderma should not stop you from having sex or being in a loving relationship. But it may take some work. If you and your partner are both feeling isolated and are having problems working out your feelings, get help. Your physician can be an excellent resource. If you feel uncomfortable discussing sexual matters with your doctors (many do), you do have other options. You may want to give couples therapy a try. Or even sex therapy. Whatever the answer is for you, just make sure you and your partner are working together toward a mutually agreeable solution. We all need intimacy in our lives. Don't let scleroderma take that away from you too.

IN A SENTENCE:

> *Even though you may have to make some changes, you can still enjoy a loving and intimate relationship with your partner.*

learning

Is Pregnancy
an Option for You?

SO . . . YOU want to have a baby. Only now you've been saddled with this lifelong disease and are wondering if your dreams will ever become a reality. Deciding to have a baby is an enormous decision to make, even when you're healthy. But it becomes especially complicated when your ill health is factored into the equation. If you have the localized form of scleroderma, rest assured your condition does *not* present a higher than normal risk during pregnancy. But if you have the systemic form, many things must be taken into consideration before you become pregnant. In the past, women with the systemic form of scleroderma were often advised not to become pregnant. The good news is, that advice is changing. Thanks to improved medical treatments, as well as a better understanding of the disease itself, many women have gone on to have successful pregnancies and healthy babies. However, each woman's case is unique; a decision to have a baby should be made only after considering all the risks involved.

Should I or shouldn't I?

When you are contemplating pregnancy, every aspect of your disease becomes a factor. From disease duration to medications being taken, every issue must be thoroughly evaluated with your physician prior to making your decision. Some of the most important factors to consider include the following:

1. ***Disease duration***—Most scleroderma experts agree that if a patient has been diagnosed with systemic disease, she should wait at least two to three years before becoming pregnant. Not only does this give the disease time to stabilize, but it also gives the doctor a better idea of how severe the disease is and what organs have been affected.
2. ***Limited versus diffuse disease***—Although patients with limited disease incur less risk than those with diffuse disease, each disease type presents its own set of possible complications. Those with limited disease run the risk of blood pressure and kidney problems; those with diffuse disease run the risk of blood pressure problems, kidney disease, and heart disease.
3. ***Current medications***—Because of the possible damage to the baby, most medications must be stopped prior to becoming pregnant. Some drug classes can be substituted for other, less-powerful medications (like antacids for proton pump inhibitors, if you have reflux); other drug classes can't be so easily changed. If you're dependent on a lot of medications to control your symptoms, this is just one more reason to wait until your disease has stabilized before you become pregnant.

Will it be harder to conceive?

In a study on pregnancy in women with scleroderma conducted by Virginia Steen, professor of medicine at Georgetown University, the results suggested that overall, scleroderma patients did not have reduced fertility. However, be aware that some of the medications used in the treatment of scleroderma can contribute to infertility. Two medications are particular culprits: prednisone (or other types of steroids) and Cytoxan (cyclophosphamide). Prednisone, along with all its other nasty side effects, can cause menstrual irregularities as well as decreased fertility. Cytoxan can cause the onset of early menopause. If your condition necessitates the use of Cytoxan and you know you'd like to become pregnant down the road, speak to your doctor about ways to help you protect your fertility. But you must do this prior to starting the medication and realize ahead of time that nothing is guaranteed. Another option would be to speak to your doctor about the possibility of using a less toxic medication in lieu of Cytoxan. Keep in mind, you may not have a choice of medications to use if your physician feels that an organ is being threatened and that Cytoxan is the best and only treatment for you. Remember, *your* life should always come first.

Pregnancy management

While many women with scleroderma can safely have healthy pregnancies, the pregnancy should be considered a high-risk pregnancy and followed by a physician specializing in high-risk pregnancies (perinatologist). Ideally, this physician should work closely with the other members of your medical team to ensure both your safety and the baby's. The good news is that the results of Steen's study also showed that there was no increase in the rate of miscarriage among scleroderma patients except in those with long-standing diffuse disease. Other findings from the study show an improvement in certain symptoms like Raynaud's phenomenon, but a worsening of GI symptoms such as reflux. And for those patients who had experienced renal crisis prior to becoming pregnant, the results of the study were also positive. It seems those patients with renal problems all had healthy babies even while taking ACE inhibitors, a drug required to control blood pressure after renal crisis. A word of caution if you depend on ACE inhibitors to control your blood pressure and want to become pregnant: Because ACE inhibitors are associated with severe kidney problems in the baby, every attempt should be made to control blood pressure with medications other than ACE inhibitors. However, the reality is that the risks to the mother with uncontrolled **hypertension** (high blood pressure) are much higher than the risks to the baby. The bottom line for renal patients: You must do whatever possible to make sure your blood pressure is controlled during your pregnancy, even if it means taking ACE inhibitors.

More good news for renal patients comes out of a separate study on pregnancy, also done by Steen, which showed that none of the babies of mothers who continued on ACE inhibitors during their pregnancies were born with any kidney problems.

Is there a predictable course for pregnancy in scleroderma?

Although studies have shown that there is a higher incidence both of premature infants and of smaller (low birth weight) full-term infants among the scleroderma population, the pregnancy course and outcome of any one individual cannot be predicted. Consider the following patients' experiences: Kathryn was diagnosed with diffuse disease during her pregnancy. Although her disease seemed to peak in activity during her pregnancy and she developed sclerosis of the placenta, she went on to deliver a healthy six-pound, two-ounce baby three weeks early. Beverly, on the other hand, developed fluid in her lungs and had to have an emergency cesarean. She delivered a five-pound, nine-ounce baby four weeks early who unfortunately had multiple health problems at birth. Ironically, her disease settled down after her pregnancy. Another scleroderma patient spoke of a problem-free pregnancy and delivered a full-term, healthy baby. Three patients, three different experiences. It's nice to have facts and statistics, but the reality is that there is no way to predict what any one particular patient's experience with pregnancy will be. The best you can do is to have both your disease and your pregnancy monitored regularly and remain optimistic.

The decision to become pregnant must be an informed one

When you have a chronic disease, the decision to have a baby is not an easy one. Not only do you have the normal issues to consider, such as your age, family, and financial situation, but you also have to think about how your disease will impact your pregnancy. There is no easy answer; the decision to become pregnant is as individualized as your disease. Many patients go on to have successful pregnancies and healthy babies, but others are not so lucky. Then there are patients who feel the risks of a pregnancy are too great to their health and decide against it. There is no right or wrong decision; there is only the decision that's right for you. Just make sure you've considered your options and are aware of both the risks and the benefits involved.

IN A SENTENCE:

> *Pregnancy in a scleroderma patient with systemic disease is considered high-risk and requires careful monitoring of both the disease and the pregnancy.*

Stress and Your Disease

YOU KNOW the feeling: racing heartbeat, pulsing blood, tensed muscles, queasy stomach, sweaty hands. It's called the stress response, the body's hormonal reaction to protect itself against any real or perceived threats. Also referred to as the "fight or flight" response, it lets us know that, on some level, something's wrong. All these physical reactions were designed to save your life. But, if the stress response is sustained for extended periods of time, the stress response itself can become a threat to your body, by leaving the body always on "alert." And that can exacerbate your disease.

In today's society, stress seems to be a four-letter word. People will go to great lengths to try to avoid it and are willing to try just about anything to get rid of it. But stress itself isn't necessarily a bad thing—it's all in how you handle it. All of us have different stress tolerance levels. There are those who thrive on it; others are paralyzed by it. And there are different kinds of stress. Stress can be acute (brought on by a specific event) or chronic (lasting a long time). Acute stress can be handled pretty quickly; chronic stress may take more time and/or lifestyle changes. Everybody handles stress differently. The key is to determine your personal tolerance for stress.

Stress can make you sick(er)

High levels of stress can make you sick, period. Not only are high levels of stress associated with increased heart disease risks, such as high blood pressure and high cholesterol levels, there is evidence of its role in gastrointestinal, dermatological, emotional, and respiratory ailments, as well. Stress is also linked to immune system disturbances, leaving many susceptible to colds, coughs, and infections. It can also destroy the immunological balance of your digestive and urinary systems, leading to an overgrowth of harmful bacteria. And wait, there's more. Other bodily reactions to stress include headaches, chest pain, muscle tension, hives or skin rashes, high blood pressure, indigestion, increased sweating, insomnia, constipation, diarrhea, shortness of breath, loss of appetite, and a dry throat. And then there's the emotional reaction to stress, such as irritability, anger, hypersensitivity, apathy, and depression. Obviously, not everybody gets all of these stress-related symptoms. But who wants *any* of them? The important thing is to identify the things in your life that are most stressful to you and try to eliminate them as best as possible. You have enough health problems right now. Don't let the stress in your life contribute to more health problems than you can handle.

Stress and your disease

If the above information isn't enough to convince you to try to eliminate the stress in your life, consider this: Stress has been fingered as the culprit in flare-ups of both arthritis and asthma, and evidence has also shown that certain animals with autoimmune disease have a defective hormone neuron (**corticotropin-releasing hormone**—made in the hypothalamus) that accelerates inflammation under stressful situations. Stress can also aggravate your symptoms by releasing chemicals that can cause fatigue. High levels of stress can also lead to unhealthy lifestyle habits, such as cigarettes, drugs, and alcohol. The bottom line? Who needs more inflammation and fatigue? Stress can exacerbate your symptoms and wreak havoc on your disease.

Laugh it off

Want a treatment that's painless, free, and fun? Go ahead and laugh. No, really. Chortle, chuckle, giggle, guffaw—whichever you do, just let 'er rip. Odds are you'll feel better afterward. Laughing allows you to boost your immune system, ease your pain, relax your body, and reduce your stress hormones. And it's free.

Although the first studies of the effect of humor on the body were conducted in the 1930s, the most intriguing findings came much later, from studies conducted at Loma Linda University School of Medicine in California. They found that when students watched funny videos, they had a significant increase in **T cells** and natural killer cells, both of which fight off diseases. It was also discovered that the students had lower levels of the stress hormone **cortisol** in their blood.

In another study, conducted by the Oakhurst Health Research Institute in California, it was discovered that first-time heart attack sufferers who spent thirty minutes a day chortling at comedy videos were less likely to have a second heart attack.

Although more studies are needed, one thing is clear: Laughter promotes wellness and healing. So when you're feeling stressed, go ahead and laugh. There's no better way to release those endorphins and experience laughter's healing effects.

Stress management

Not only will decreasing the stress in your life increase your energy, it will lift your outlook. There are many different ways to help manage your stress; find the way that works for you. Consider the following:

1. **Learn to say no.** You may be taking on more responsibility than you should. Eliminate any activities that aren't absolutely necessary in your life. This may mean modifying your job description or changing some of your responsibilities at home. It's okay to delegate.
2. **Accept your limitations.** Your life is different now. You have a chronic illness. Don't expect yourself to be able to do everything you were able to do before your diagnosis. And don't be afraid to ask for help if you need it.

3. **Allow yourself to relax every day.** Whether it's listening to music, reading a good book, painting a picture, or watching a movie, make time in your daily schedule to focus on just yourself. Other ideas include

   ○ meditation
   ○ visualization
   ○ deep breathing excercises
   ○ aromatherapy
   ○ massage
   ○ tai chi
   ○ biofeedback
   ○ yoga

4. **Get some exercise.** Exercise is one of the best stress relievers around. Physical activity benefits not only your body, but your mind as well.

5. **Allow yourself to cry.** Just as laughing can relieve stress, so can crying. Forget the social stigma attached. Feel free to shed your tears when you feel the need. Tears are a natural way for the body to reduce anxiety, release negative feelings, and recharge your emotions. A good cry almost always causes emotional relief.

6. **Don't neglect your diet.** Anxiety and stress can cause you to neglect proper eating habits. Some people overeat when under stress; others forget to eat. Don't binge or skip any meals. You'll only feel worse. Try to make sure your diet is as consistent as possible.

7. **Make sure you get a good night's sleep.** Getting enough rest is key to staying healthy. Lack of sleep lowers your immunity and aggravates your disease process.

8. **Talk about your feelings.** Whether it's with a therapist, rabbi, priest, friend, family member, or coworker, share your feelings. It's unhealthy to keep them bottled up. You don't need to cope alone. Because you're not alone.

9. **Take it a day at a time.** Try to live in the moment. Don't let yourself feel overwhelmed by long to-do lists. And try not to feel like you have to get everything done at once. Pace yourself. Do one task at a

time. Give it your full attention; once it's completed, go on to the next. Remember, there's always tomorrow.

The reality of stress

Let's face it. The diagnosis of a chronic disease is stressful. It can leave you feeling powerless and out of control, not to mention emotionally drained. And that can challenge your ability to cope. As I mentioned earlier, when your body is worn down from the illness itself, you can be even more susceptible to stress. That can wreak havoc on your disease. Although certain types of stress may be unavoidable, the key is to find stress-management tools that work for you.

IN A SENTENCE:

> *Try not to let your stress exacerbate your disease symptoms: Develop a healthy and realistic attitude toward stress, and identify the things that are most stressful to you.*

learning

Your Health Comes First, Period

IF YOU'RE anything like me, remembering to put your health first takes a lot of practice. But then again, I have a Jewish mother who keeps reminding me—for which I'm eternally grateful. In the beginning, when your disease is still new, it may seem like all you're doing is putting your health first. Your entire life is focused on your disease and everything else in your life seems to take a backseat. But as time goes on and you begin to understand more about how your disease is going to affect your life, things may begin to change. You start to live your life normally again and begin to focus on other things besides your health. In fact, after living with scleroderma for the last ten months, you may have already reached that point. Now comes the trickier part. You probably thought you had gotten through the hardest part: your diagnosis. Now you realize you face something even more daunting: learning to live day in and day out with scleroderma.

The importance of putting your health first

Now, don't get me wrong. I'm all for leading an active, full life. Just not at the expense of my health. Say, for example, you promised to take your kids to Disneyland over the summer vacation. You've been planning the excursion for several months and your kids have been talking nonstop about it. Unfortunately, as the day approaches, you find yourself feeling unusually tired and know you don't feel quite right. When the day finally arrives, you're feeling horrible. But you're riddled with guilt. You don't want to let your kids down, yet you can hardly get out of bed. What do you do?

○ **Scenario 1:** You drag yourself out of bed and decide you're going to go. You hardly have enough energy to get yourself ready, let alone your kids. On the drive down to Disneyland, you're caught in a traffic jam; your drive is an hour longer than normal. The kids are fighting in the backseat and you begin to feel incredibly anxious and irritable. And, you're beginning to realize you've made the wrong decision and wish you had stayed home. You finally get to Disneyland and you're already exhausted. Then come the crowds, the long lines, the hot weather—things that are hard enough to deal with even on a good day. You make it through the day only to get home and collapse. Your excursion has worn you out so much, you're in bed for the next three days. You end up having to hire a babysitter to watch the kids as you're just not up to it yet. Then you think, if you'd only listened to your body, you would've been in bed for one day instead of three.

○ **Scenario 2:** You decide to stay in bed and have a heart-to-heart talk with your kids. You explain how you're feeling and how disappointed you are at not being able to take them to Disneyland. You promise to go another day and plan another date right then and there. Then you take them to the video store, get a few of their favorite videos, make some popcorn, and get back in bed. You spend the rest of the day resting, and by the next day you're feeling much better. You're then able to spend some quality time with your kids and everybody's happy.

When you don't put you and your health first, nobody wins. I know. I have experienced both of the above scenarios. And after learning the hard way, as in Scenario 1, I finally realized that if I don't put my health first, I am not only not being fair to myself, I'm not being fair to my family, either.

Listening to your body

Even though you may feel like your body has betrayed you by getting a disease, you must make peace with it. Now, more than ever, you're going to have to befriend your body and listen to what it's telling you. And that may take some time and some hard-earned lessons like the one above. When you weren't feeling well before your diagnosis, you probably just pushed through it until you began to feel better. At least, that's what I did. Not so, after my diagnosis. I couldn't just "push through it" anymore, because if I did, I'd suffer the consequences. If I pushed myself too hard, that meant spending several extra days in bed. Now, I listen to my body. At the first sign of any trouble, I stop and rest—for however long it takes until I feel better. This way, I'm up and about in a much shorter period of time, instead of pushing myself to exhaustion and having to take that much more time to recover from it.

Pace yourself

This brings us to a very important topic: learning to pace yourself. You've learned the value of pacing yourself throughout this book and now we're going to focus on it again. You have a new priority in your life, your health, and as is often the case with new priorities, you're going to need to shift some of your other priorities around to make room for this new one. That shifting may take some time to learn how to do. Shifting around your priorities also entails the possibility of having to change, which can be very difficult. But you must do whatever it takes to make your health your number-one priority. And this includes pacing yourself in your everyday life. To learn more about how to pace yourself, ask yourself the following questions:

1. Are you trying to get too much done in one day?
2. Is your job causing you excess stress and fatigue?

3. Do you have a hard time saying no?
4. Do you feel the need to get everything done on your own?
5. Do people often tell you you're like superwoman?
6. Are you having a hard time keeping up with the housework?
7. Is your personal life stretched too thin?

If you answered "yes" to the above questions, you're not pacing yourself. Consider the following suggestions to help you learn how to pace yourself:

○ Stop worrying about your to-do list. Break it up into smaller lists. Don't put unrealistic expectations on yourself to get it all done today. Only do what you absolutely have to get done. Remember, there's always tomorrow.

○ If your job is eating up all your good energy and putting your health at risk, you need to reassess your options. Ask about job-sharing or working part-time.

○ You must incorporate the word "no" into your vocabulary. And the sooner the better.

○ You don't have to do everything on your own. Delegate some of your responsibilities to others. Like your kids. Or your coworkers. You'd be surprised how many people are willing to help. You just have to learn how to ask.

○ Who wants to be superwoman when all it means is spending most of your free time feeling sick in bed?

○ What's more important, having clean windows or feeling well?

○ You need to be able to put yourself first. Having lots of friends is wonderful, but not at the expense of your health. Good friends will understand. And if they don't, they certainly don't have your best interests at heart.

Start now

Putting your health first is not an option, it's a necessity. Although it may feel awkward at first, in time you will get used to it. Like all new things, putting your health first may take some practice. But once you get the hang of it, it becomes second nature. And you'll be surprised at the difference it can make in how you feel in your life. Find the Jewish mother in your life who can give you a gentle reminder every now and then. Your health should always come first. Your well-being depends on it and your long-term health is counting on it.

IN A SENTENCE:

> *When you have a chronic disease like scleroderma, your health needs to be your first priority.*

Is Your Life Working for You?

YOU'VE BEEN living with your disease for almost a year now and are thinking about how far you've come. Some of you may have breezed right through the year; others haven't been so lucky and have had to struggle day by day. You think back to the early days of your diagnosis and feel relieved that you've made it to this point. Nevertheless, something still doesn't feel right. You're not quite sure where the feeling's coming from, but it keeps gnawing at you. And finally, it comes to you: Your old life, as you know it, no longer exists. You've been living a new life this past year but you haven't had the time to figure out how to live it. You've been so bogged down in the day-to-day minutiae of living with a chronic disease, you've yet to discover what's working for you in this new life and what's not. Until now, that is. You took stock of your medical world in Month 8; now it's time to take stock of the rest of your world and reexamine your new life.

Where to begin

Reexamining your life does not mean overhauling your entire life. You've already done that, just by getting a chronic disease.

Reexamining simply means assessing what's working for you and what's not, with the ultimate goal of achieving a more balanced life. You'll read more about ideas on how to achieve that balance in the Learning section of this chapter. In the meantime, you may want to take out a pencil and paper and begin to list all the different areas in your life: work, family, health, children, hobbies, friends, fitness, diet, travel, and whatever else you consider to be an important part of your life. Now, put a check mark next to those areas of your life that may not be working as well as you'd like. Next, think about what you'd like to change in that particular area; jot down a few ideas. We'll talk about implementing those ideas later in the chapter.

Why it's important to reexamine your life

In the Learning section of Month 10, you learned the importance of putting your health first; the act of rebalancing your life will allow you to do just that. When my doctor told me something had to give in my life or my health would continue to suffer, I tried to downplay the importance of his words. But as my health continued to deteriorate, it became apparent that it was finally time to take his advice seriously. My life at that time was stretched pretty thin between work, family, and my health. In my quest to do it all, I wasn't being fair to anybody in my life, including myself. After quite a bit of soul searching, I sat down and made a list like the one outlined above. Afterward, I was surprised at how out of balance my life felt to me. I then began taking the necessary steps to make some changes in my life. Was it difficult? Absolutely. Was it worth it? Without a doubt. The changes I was able to make allowed me to better focus on my health and my family, and as a result lead a better-balanced, more enriching life.

Is your life lopsided?

It's no surprise to anyone that when you begin to place too much emphasis on any one particular area of your life, other areas of your life begin to suffer. Take the workaholic, for example. Odds are that person is spending so much time at work that his or her family life may be falling apart. A single workaholic probably has no personal life whatsoever. And just the opposite can be true, as well: When you're focused on too many things at once, like I was, you're pulled in a million different directions and can't focus very well on any one thing in particular. Sometimes it takes something drastic, like a serious health problem, to make you realize your life is out of balance and that you need to be true to yourself first. Now that you've been diagnosed with scleroderma, it's time to make some changes. Maybe you've been focusing too much on your disease this past year and you need to take a step back to gain some perspective. Or, perhaps you've been neglecting your health because you've been in denial ever since your diagnosis. Whatever your particular situation, it's time to sit back and ask yourself if your life is working for you the way it is right now. If it is, congratulations. You've succeeded in keeping your life on track in spite of your disease. But for the rest of you, it's time to sit back and do some serious renegotiating with yourselves.

When new plans go awry

While there's never a good time to get a disease, the timing of your diagnosis can really wreak havoc on your life. Maybe you had just started a new job or were thinking about starting a family. Well, you know what they say about the best-laid plans. But just because you got a new disease doesn't mean you can't accomplish these things. It's just a matter of timing. Remember, you can make your life work for you. If you need to, take the time to deal with your disease before you start that new job or begin your family. Your health needs to be your first priority right now. Ask your new employer if you can take a short leave of absence until you can get your health situation under control. If your employer says no, consider yourself lucky to have found out early on how inflexible he or she is. After all, you have a chronic disease; this will not be the only time you'll need to take some time off. Same thing goes for starting your family. You found out in the Learning section of Month 9 the importance of waiting until your disease stabilizes (if you have the systemic form) before becoming pregnant. Optimally, you'd like to bring a child into this world when you're at your healthiest—for both you and your baby.

You're on the right track

Many patients think the first year is the hardest, and the good news is, it's almost over. You've had to learn how to live your life in the best way you could while incorporating a new disease into your daily living. Reexamining your life at this point allows you to move forward knowing you've done everything possible to make sure your life is working the way you want it to. That doesn't mean you can't reassess your life again in another year or even in six months. In fact, doing so guarantees you'll be closer to living the life you choose. Whether it means quitting your job, changing your diet, taking a vacation, or just focusing on you and your health, your life will work better because you're the one in control of it.

IN A SENTENCE:

> *If your life isn't working the way you'd like it to right now, you must make the necessary changes to live the life you want.*

learning

Achieving Balance in Your Life

YOU LEARNED the value of reexamining your life in the Living section of this chapter; now we're going to talk about how to achieve some much-needed balance in your life. And this may mean changing some parts of your life. Oops, I said it: C-H-A-N-G-E. For some, change can be a welcome necessity, but for others, change can be a dirty word evoking tremendous fear and anxiety. When people become fearful of change, it can often cause a sense of paralysis that prevents them from taking any positive steps forward in their lives. If change causes that sort of reaction for you, that's okay. There's a way to go about change that can make it feel a lot less intimidating, even tolerable. It's all in how you approach it. You learned earlier in the chapter that when one particular area of your life gets all your attention, other areas can begin to suffer. And before you know it, your life becomes out of balance. Let's talk about ways to restructure your current life with the goal of reducing stress, eliminating baggage, refocusing on the positives in your life, and learning to enjoy the moment. After all, isn't that what life's all about?

Yes, you are in control of your life

Now, don't get me wrong. Learning to rebalance your life is no easy task. Especially when you feel as if you've lost control over your life because of your new disease. But remember: *You are in control.* It may not seem like it, but you have much more control over your life now than ever before. Why? Because you've learned the value of your health. And although it was probably one of the toughest lessons you've ever learned, hopefully you've gained a new appreciation for what's important in your life. As is often said, adversity only makes us stronger. But the cost of rebalancing your life often means making some hard choices. And those choices usually involve change. With that said, let's talk about the meaning of change.

To change or not to change

Change, as defined by *Webster's New World Dictionary,* means **1.** to put or take in place of something else, **2.** to exchange, **3.** to make different, alter, **4.** a substitution, alteration or variation. Sounds easy enough, right? That depends on how you feel about change. Sometimes the changes you need to make in your life are monumental; others are slight. Some are easy to make, some are more difficult. But if you keep focusing on finding that equilibrium in your life, the changes you have to make to achieve that balance won't seem so overwhelming. Especially if you don't make the changes all at once. There are many different areas in your life that can be tweaked to find just the right amount of balance you need. But where do you start? Below is a list of questions about the different areas of your life that you may need to reevaluate. Think about the amount of physical and emotional energy you spend in each area, and contemplate any changes that you may need to make to feel better about that particular area of your life. If you're the type who doesn't respond well to change, take baby steps. For instance, say you want to begin an exercise program but the thought of it fills you with dread. Because of your disease, you haven't been able to exercise much this past year and are now completely out of shape. This is the time to think small. Before you decide to join a gym, which can overwhelm even the most active of us, start out with something smaller, like a walk around your neighborhood, or a gentle swim in a pool. Then, when you become more comfortable with your new routine, step up the pace. You may even want to set a small goal for yourself. But if the thought of not reaching that goal is more stressful than the exercise program itself, forget it. Remember, you have only yourself to please. Don't make the changes any harder than they have to be. Your goal is to achieve more balance in your life, not more stress.

Ways to help you achieve more balance

It's time to ask yourself the following questions:

1. **Is your job less than satisfying?** Or, is your health suffering because of your job? If so, it's time to reevaluate your needs. If your job is just a means to an end, it's time for a change. Reread the Living section of Month 4 to help you make the changes that will allow you to achieve the balance you're looking for.
2. **Are you spending enough time with your family and friends?** Has your disease made you feel more isolated and less interested in spending time with your friends and family? If so, it's time to change. Don't avoid the very thing that you might need the most right now. Those closest to you can offer you strength and support. And they can rejuvenate your spirit. Family and friends make us feel grounded. But if you find your family has the opposite effect on you, focus on those in your life who do provide you with the type of love and support you need right now.
3. **Are you getting enough exercise?** Not only is exercise a great stress reliever, it's a necessity for your health. Everybody needs exercise, even those with a chronic disease. You don't have to start by running a marathon. But you do have to start. Start small and do only what you're comfortable doing. And most importantly, always check with your doctor before you start any type of exercise program.
4. **Do you have hobbies you enjoy?** Sometimes when life gets so busy, we neglect the things that bring us pleasure. Or, perhaps you're unable to do what you used to do because of changes in your hands, or your overwhelming fatigue. That's okay. You need to find other things that can bring you pleasure. Not only are hobbies good for your emotional health, they're a nice diversion from dealing with the daily rigors of a chronic disease.

5. ***Have you taken a vacation lately?*** Travel can revive and refresh our spirit and restore our sanity. You don't have to go to a tropical island to get the benefits. Whether it's a day, a weekend, or longer, a change of pace and scenery can often be just the thing you need to restore your sense of balance in the world. Just make sure to pack your meds and don't overdo it. I guarantee you'll come back wishing you had gone sooner.

6. ***Have you ever thought about volunteering?*** Volunteering is a wonderful way to look beyond ourselves and focus on others. Not only does it give you a wonderful sense of purpose, it can also give you a new perspective on your own problems. If you think you're not ready to make that big a commitment or you're worried about how your health will be affected by adding one more thing to your busy life, don't be. The good news about volunteering is that you can put in as much time or as little time as you want. The choice is yours. Even if you can't go into an office, many organizations can still find things for you to do at home, like helping out with a mailing, or making phone calls. Once you get involved, I think you'll find volunteering to be a very rich and rewarding experience.

7. ***Is spirituality important to you?*** If so, you need to make an effort to incorporate more spirituality into your life. Whether you join a temple or a church, make an effort to pray more, or do something as simple as daily meditation, find that something special that's meaningful to you. Remember, spirituality is free. You have nothing to lose. Nothing ventured, nothing gained.

8. ***Do you enjoy animals?*** Studies have shown that those who own pets are less stressed than those who don't. Interaction with a pet has been found to lower cortisol levels as well as increase serotonin levels. Pets are loyal, nonjudgmental, good listeners, and are always happy to see you. Although it adds another responsibility to your life, I think you'll find the rewards of owning a pet far outweigh the burdens.

9. ***Have you spent any time alone lately?*** Obligations to others in your life can be mentally draining. Sometimes all it takes for you to recharge your batteries is spending some time alone with yourself. See a movie, take a walk, go to a museum, or just sit down with a good book. Just make sure the focus is on you and you only. You'll be amazed at how refreshed you feel afterward.

10. *Is it time to reevaluate the relationships in your life?* Relationships, like good food, can get stale. It's time to get rid of the ones in your life that are too draining and too much trouble. If you're like me, you hardly have time in your life for those people you want to see, let alone those you don't. Don't waste what little personal time you have on relationships that aren't working. While it may seem a bit harsh to "clean house" in the beginning, you'll be glad you did in the long run.

11. *How's your nutrition?* We all know a sensible diet is essential to our good health. But eating right often is not as easy as it sounds. If changing your diet has been on your to-do list for longer than you'd like to admit, now's the time to make that change. Eating the wrong foods may be contributing to a lack of energy or listlessness. If you need to, see a nutritionist. Oftentimes when you make a financial commitment, the psychological commitment follows. Start today and you'll be surprised at how much better you feel tomorrow.

12. *Is it time to clean out the clutter in your life?* Sick of looking at the same old clothes that have been in your closet for the last ten years? Or the extra bedroom in your house that has become the "storage" room? And what about your car? Found any old parking tickets under the seats lately? If you answered yes to any of these questions, it's time to start cleaning out the clutter. You'll feel a renewed sense of space and freedom afterward. And at the very least, you'll have created new space for that extra-special something you just couldn't live without.

There may be other areas of your life not mentioned above that you may find need reexamining as well. Each person's priorities are different, but the process is the same. Now that you've learned the value of your health, finding the balance you need in your life may be a lot easier. And that leads to a happier and healthier life overall.

IN A SENTENCE:

> *Achieving balance in our lives comes from reexamining our priorities and reshaping their value.*

MONTH **12**

Getting on with Life

YOU'VE MADE it. It's been a year since you were first diagnosed and you've come a long way. Congratulations. Now, take a minute to think back to when you were first diagnosed. Do you remember where you were in your life? It probably felt as if your whole world had stopped. Certain parts of your life were put on hold. You've spent quite a bit of time this past year focused on scleroderma and the changes you've had to make to accommodate your new disease; now it's time to look forward. Life goes on. And if there's one thing you probably learned this past year, it's that life is short and you need to make the most of every minute of it.

Moving forward

Most of you are thrilled to have made it through your first year, but some may feel a bit gun-shy about moving forward. After all, you've been through a life-changing event and you're just now beginning to get your bearings. You learned in Month 11 how to reexamine your life to achieve the balance you need. Now that you've achieved that balance, you're probably asking yourself, How do I move forward living with an unpredictable disease? How will I know what to expect? These are normal questions to be asking yourself. And the answer is twofold. If you can, try and pick up your life right where you left off. Metaphorically speaking, of course. Obviously, many things in your life may be different now. You may have had to change your job. Or you may not be able to do the same things you were once able to do. But you can try to incorporate those changes into your new life and continue on your original path. It may not be exactly what you had in mind or how you had planned it, but that's okay. Living with a chronic disease means learning to be flexible. And always having a Plan B.

Another option is to look at this experience as an opportunity to start over. Maybe you were at a crossroads in your life when you were diagnosed and weren't quite sure in which direction your life was headed. One scleroderma patient I know had always dreamed of starting a business out of her home. She was working at a dead-end job and wanted to be able to spend more time with her kids. Sure enough, shortly after she was diagnosed, she was forced to quit her job and was able to start a small business out of her kitchen. While she wasn't thrilled at the reason for having to make the change, she couldn't believe she was actually living her dream. It's the ol' "making lemonade out of lemons" scenario. Sometimes good things do come out of bad experiences. But you need to know where to look for them.

As for not knowing what to expect in your life, well, who does? We all live with a certain amount of uncertainty every day—disease or no disease. And while having a disease certainly enhances that uncertainty, don't use it as an excuse to not live your life the way you want to—albeit with a few extra compromises.

"But, you look so well . . ."

While the majority of scleroderma patients experience physical changes in their appearance that are noticeable to others, some don't. The fact is, many autoimmune diseases are hidden diseases. And this can make it difficult when moving forward with your life. For those patients who don't suffer any visible changes in appearance, many people unfamiliar with the disease will have a hard time believing there's anything wrong with you. And even those who are familiar with scleroderma often don't fully understand the realities of the disease. I can't count the number of times I've heard, "But, you look so well," during times when I've felt my worst. And I remember thinking to myself, "That's a relief, because if I looked as bad as I felt then I'd really be in trouble." But although it's not such a bad thing to look okay when you're not, problems can arise from other people's expectations of you. Don't ever do something when you don't feel up to it just because of someone else's expectation of you. Or because you look well. You're the one who will ultimately pay for it. As you begin to move forward, don't let others' insensitivity get the best of you. Learn to trust your instincts. You've been living with the disease long enough to know its ups and downs. Always do what's best for you no matter how you feel or what you look like.

Keep your sense of humor

While there's nothing funny about getting scleroderma, maintaining a sense of humor throughout your journey will take you a long way. No journey is without some amusement. Although certain things may not seem particularly funny when they happen, sometimes when you get some distance or look at it from a different perspective, you'll see things differently. That's what happened to me. Shortly after I was diagnosed, I had to have a heart test called a transesophageal-echocardiogram. The procedure involves having a scope put down your esophagus to get a better look at your heart. The worst part about taking the test is having to swallow the scope *before* you're actually put under. For weeks beforehand, I panicked just thinking about that part of the test. I kept thinking, What if I can't swallow it or what happens if I can't stop gagging? Worse yet, what happens if I vomit all over my doctor?! I nearly drove myself crazy thinking about it. Ironically, I wasn't the least bit worried about the actual results of the test, just the procedure itself. Go figure. When the day of the test arrived, I made sure to let the nurses know about my fear of swallowing the scope. Obviously, I wasn't the first patient to feel this way. But they couldn't have been nicer about it and gently walked me through every step of the "swallowing." And it worked. I actually did it, I swallowed the scope. I was so relieved. The doctor finally arrived to begin the test having had no idea about my earlier anxiety of the dreaded scope. About halfway through the test, I heard my doctor begin to swear. Alarmed, I bolted up off the table thinking he'd found something horribly wrong with my heart. But no, it wasn't my heart. It was the machine needed to do the procedure. It had decided to stop working right in the middle of my test. Then panic struck me: Was I actually going to have to *re-do* the test, swallowing and all? Yep— you guessed it. We had to start from square one, which meant having to go through the whole scope swallowing thing one more time. Being so doped up at that point, the scope went down without a hitch. (Why couldn't they have done that the first time around?!) But my doctor said he's never seen a machine break in the twenty years he'd been doing this procedure. And while it was tough to see the humor in it while it was happening, I couldn't help but chuckle with my nurses afterward. Of all people to have this happen to. Even my doctor was laughing about it.

Many such incidents have occurred throughout my journey but I try to see the lighter side of these incidents. Hopefully, you too will be able to maintain your sense of humor throughout your journey. After all, what's life without laughter?

Remaining vigilant

Even though you're moving on with your life, you still must remain a vigilant patient. Scleroderma can take many twists and turns, so you always need to be prepared. Make sure to keep up with all your doctor appointments and any medical tests ordered. And don't forget to take your medication, too. Even if you're feeling better. Scleroderma may have changed your life, but that doesn't mean you can't move on and live a fulfilling life. Be as positive as you can while making plans for your future. Now, go and get on with the rest of your life.

IN A SENTENCE:

> *You've survived your first year of scleroderma; now it's time to move forward and live your life as best you can.*

learning

Living Well with Scleroderma ... Really

THERE'S NO denying that getting scleroderma is a life-changing event. And you've probably spent most of your life this last year focused on learning how to cope with this life-changing event. Now it's time to put your new coping skills to the test. It's time to move forward and continue to fulfill your hopes and dreams. Don't know where to start? Look inward. As we've navigated together through your first year with scleroderma, there's one last thing we haven't covered yet. And that's hope. With it, we have the power within us to live each day to the fullest and appreciate every moment we have. Without it, we lose our perspective on life and sometimes feel as if we don't have much to live for. Hope allows us to achieve our goals and realize our dreams. And it allows us to be positive about the future.

The pursuit of happiness

Scleroderma may not have been in your five-year plan, but that doesn't mean you have to forgo the plans that were. Your plans may need a little tweaking now, but you should make every effort to fulfill them. Living your life well and living your life with a chronic disease aren't mutually exclusive. The pursuit of happiness is the same whether you're healthy or ill. Dealing with adversity can create unforeseen opportunities. Let scleroderma be the impetus in your life to promote positive change. Use it as a tool to strengthen the relationships in your life. Learn to appreciate each day as it comes. Take more time for you and your family. Plant a new garden. Go back to school. Buy that new house. Get a pet. Take that new job. Start a new exercise program. Learn a new language. Go to a tropical island. Volunteer. Do whatever it is that makes you happy. Because now, more than ever, you need to find that one source of happiness to give you hope for the future.

Reviewing the Basics

AS YOU continue to move forward, sometimes it's helpful to review some of the basics you've learned along the way. In your personal quest to live well with your new disease, keep reminding yourself of the following:

- ○ Getting scleroderma is not your fault.
- ○ You're not alone.
- ○ You didn't do anything wrong.
- ○ There is no one "right" way to cope with your disease.
- ○ Keep educating yourself.
- ○ Knowledge is power.
- ○ You're in control.
- ○ Get involved in your local scleroderma community.
- ○ One person *can* make a difference.
- ○ Live each day to the fullest.
- ○ Always put your health first.
- ○ Never give up hope.

Don't let your disease define who you are

In living your life, try not to let your disease define who you are. You may look different on the outside, but you're still the same person on the inside. Your disease is just a small part of who you are. Getting scleroderma has forced many to reevaluate their lives and their priorities—helping them to find more fulfilling and satisfying ways to live their lives. Now that you have the first year of scleroderma behind you, it's time for you to do that, too, if you haven't done so already. You've learned the necessity of putting your health first and should continue to do so as you move forward. You deserve to have the life you want to live. And although it may be different than what you had originally planned and filled with a lot more unpredictability than you would've liked, you can still live a rich and rewarding life with scleroderma.

Choosing to live well with scleroderma

Life is all about choices. And choosing how you want to live your life with scleroderma is up to you. You've learned that scleroderma doesn't define who you are as a person, but it can still influence the decisions you choose to make in your life. By choosing to live well with scleroderma, you're choosing to live your life the way you want to in spite of your disease. We all face an uncertain future. That doesn't mean we must stop living our lives. If you've chosen to live well with scleroderma, you've made the right choice. After all, living well is what life is all about.

Hope for a cure

While I'd love to be able to focus this last chapter on a cure, unfortunately we're not quite there yet. But we've certainly come a long way. There are still no treatments to stop the disease process, but tremendous progress has been made in managing the daily symptoms and complications of scleroderma. According to Philip Clements, clinical professor of medicine at UCLA, "We know much more on a molecular level than ever before about what may be happening to cause disease manifestations. And we are approaching treatment in a more scientific fashion. Breakthroughs have come through targeting specific mechanisms and molecules and we've seen much bigger payoffs in this area." In addition to disease-specific treatments, there are many promising treatments in the works for autoimmune disease in general. From gene and cellular therapies to stem cell transplantation, options like these are being investigated daily, taking us that much closer to where we need to be. The good news for scleroderma is that each year, more money is being raised for research. And disease awareness is increasing every day. Even the federal government is taking notice, increasing the amount of money given each year for scleroderma research. But we all must do our part. Don't become a complacent patient. Do your part to remain an educated and knowledgeable patient. Continue to be your own advocate. Become an advocate for the disease. Get your friends and family involved. Help raise awareness. Do some fundraising. Continue to learn. Because if we all do our part, the cure we're so feverishly in search of will undoubtedly come much sooner than later. You can count on that.

IN A SENTENCE:

> *Hope gives us strength to live well with scleroderma.*

Glossary

ANEMIA: A condition in which the blood is deficient in red blood cells and/or hemoglobin.

ANTIBODIES: Proteins made by the body's white cells of the immune system for defense against bacteria and other foreign substances.

ANTICENTROMERE ANTIBODY: An antibody directed to part of the cell's nucleus; most commonly found in limited scleroderma (CREST).

ANTINUCLEAR ANTIBODY (ANA): An antibody directed against one of many components in the nucleus of the cell.

ANTIPRUITIC: Agent used to relieve itching.

ANTI-RNP: An antibody directed against ribonucleoprotein, a nucleoprotein that contains RNA; most commonly associated with lupus and mixed connective-tissue disease.

ANTI-SSA: Also called the Ro antibody, this antibody is often associated with Sjögren's syndrome.

ANTITOPOISOMERASE ANTIBODY (ANTI-SCL-70): An antibody directed against an enzyme in the nucleus; most commonly seen in diffuse scleroderma.

AUTOIMMUNE DISEASE: A disease in which the immune system attacks the body's own tissue.

AUTOIMMUNITY: A condition in which the body produces an immune response against its own tissues.

BIOFEEDBACK: The technique of making unconscious or involuntary bodily processes perceptible to the senses in order to manipulate them by conscious mental control; has proven to be a helpful treatment for Raynaud's phenomenon.

CALCINOSIS: Calcium deposits in the skin or just below the skin.

CHRONIC GRAFT VS. HOST DISEASE: A severe rejection reaction from a matched donor's bone marrow; the donor immune system cells recognize the host body tissue as foreign and mount an immune attack on it.

CLINICAL TRIAL: A research study to test either a new drug or new uses for an existing drug.

COLLAGEN: A fibrous protein made by cells that forms the lining of organs and is the basic structural protein found in bones, cartilage, and skin.

CONTRACTURES: A permanent bending of a joint so that it loses part of the range of motion; inability to fully straighten out a joint.

CORTICOTROPIN-RELEASING HORMONE: A hormone released in a part of the hypothalamus that regulates the release of adrenocorticotropin hormone (ACTH) by the pituitary gland.

CORTISOL: A glucocorticoid that is a derivative of cortisone.

CREST: Often called limited scleroderma, it is an acronym for calcinosis, Raynaud's phenomenon, esophageal dysfunction, sclerodactyly, and telangiectasias.

CYTOKINES: A group of chemicals secreted by cells of the immune system that signal cells to perform certain actions.

EN COUP DE SABRE: A form of linear scleroderma that involves the head.

EOSINOPHILIA MYALGIA SYNDROME: A condition involving muscle pain and inflammation, nerve inflammation and an increase of eosinophils in the blood.

EOSINOPHILIC FASCIITIS: An illness that causes inflammation in the fascia, the area just beneath the skin and the fat.

FIBROMYALGIA: A pain amplification syndrome characterized by fatigue, sleeping problems, and tender points in the soft tissues; seen in as many of 15-20% of scleroderma patients.

FIBROSIS: An increase of interstitial fibrous tissue (scar tissue buildup).

GENETIC: Inherited genes and traits.

HYPERTENSION: Abnormally high arterial blood pressure.

IMMUNOSUPPRESSIVE: A very strong medication used to treat scleroderma by suppressing the immune system (i.e., Cytoxan).

INFLAMMATION: Infiltration of white blood cells into the tissues resulting in swelling, heat, and redness.

INTERSTITIAL: Situated within but not restricted to or characteristic of a particular organ or tissue (i.e., interstitial lung disease).

LINEAR SCLERODERMA: A form of localized scleroderma in which the thickened skin follows the pattern of a line on the face or down an arm or leg.

MAGNETIC RESONANCE IMAGING (MRI): A noninvasive diagnostic technique that produces computerized images of internal body tissues.

MALABSORPTION: Decreased absorption of nutrients in the bowel; in scleroderma, this is due to decreased bowel motility and bacterial overgrowth.

MICROSTOMIA: Small mouth caused by the tightening of the skin on the face.

MORPHEA SCLERODERMA: A form of localized scleroderma characterized by patches of thickened skin.

MOTILITY: The state of movement; lack of motility is most commonly seen in the GI tract in scleroderma.

OVERLAP SYNDROME: Having features of two or more diseases (i.e., scleroderma *and* lupus).

PATHOGENESIS: The origination and development of a disease.

PULMONARY HYPERTENSION: High blood pressure in the pulmonary arteries; one of the most serious complications of scleroderma.

RAYNAUD'S PHENOMENON: Color changes occurring in the hands and feet (blue, white, or red) upon exposure to cold temperatures or emotional distress; if it occurs on its own without any underlying disease process, it's called Raynaud's disease.

REFLUX: The backflow of acid from the stomach into the esophagus.

RHEUMATOLOGIST: An internal medicine specialist who has completed at least a two-year fellowship studying rheumatic diseases (all forms of arthritis and autoimmune diseases).

SCLERODACTYLY: Thickening of the skin of the fingers.

SCLERODERMA SINE SCLEROSIS: Systemic scleroderma without skin involvement.

SCLEROMYXEDEMA: A condition characterized by thickened skin on the face, head, neck, and shoulders, usually sparing the hands; it is usually associated with diabetes or with a bone marrow abnormality.

SEROTONIN: A neurotransmitter that is a powerful vasoconstrictor found in the brain.

SICCA: A condition associated with a lack of secretion.

SJÖGREN'S SYNDROME: An autoimmune condition characterized by dry mucous membranes causing dry eyes, dry mouth, and, in women, a dry vagina.

T CELLS: Lymphocytes responsible for immunologic memory; they provide cellular immunity and are the body's memory cells.

TELANGIECTASIAS: Small red spots on the skin due to the enlargement (dilitation) of small blood vessels.

TRANSDERMAL: Medication absorbed through the skin into the bloodstream.

ULCERS: Often referred to as digital ulcers or skin ulcers, these unhealed sores usually appear on the fingers, either at the tips or over the knuckles, due to poor circulation.

ULTRASOUND: A noninvasive diagnostic technique using sound waves to form a two-dimensional image for the examination and measurement of internal body structures and detection of abnormalities.

For Further Reading

Horstman, Judith, et al. *The Arthritis Foundation's Guide to Alternative Therapies.* New York: Longstreet Press, 1999.

Ganim, Barbara, *Art and Healing.* New York: Three Rivers Press, 1999

Mayes, Maureen D., M.D., *The Scleroderma Book.* New York: Oxford University Press, 1999.

Wallace, Daniel J., M.D., *The Lupus Book.* Revised and Expanded Edition. New York: Oxford University Press, 2000.

Wallace, Daniel J., M.D., and Janice Brock Wallace. *All About Fibromyalgia.* New York: Oxford University Press, 2002.

Zuckerman, Eugenia, and Julie R. Ingelfinger, M.D. *Coping with Prednisone.* New York: St. Martin's Press, 1997.

Scleroderma textbooks

Clements, Philip J., M.D. and Daniel E. Furst, M.D. *Systemic Sclerosis.* 1st ed. Philadelphia: Lippincott Williams & Wilkins, 1996.

Clements, Philip J., M.D. and Daniel E. Furst, M.D. *Systemic Sclerosis.* 2nd ed. Philadelphia: Lippincott Williams & Wilkins, 2003.

Scleroderma pamphlets

Pamphlets on all aspects of scleroderma are available in both English and Spanish from the Scleroderma Foundation, 800-722-HOPE (4673).

Resources

American Academy of Dermatology
930 E. Woodfield Road
Schaumburg, IL 60173-4927
(847) 330-0230
www.aad.org

American Autoimmune Related Diseases Association, Inc.
22100 Gratiot Avenue
E. Detroit, MI 48021-2227
(586) 776-3900
www.aarda.org

American College of Rheumatology
1800 Century Place, Suite 250
Atlanta, GA 30345
(404) 633-3777
www.rheumatology.org

Arthritis Foundation
1330 W. Peachtree Street
Atlanta, GA 30309
(800) 283-7800
www.arthritis.org

Fibromyalgia Network
PO Box 31750
Tucson, AZ 85751
(800) 853-2929
www.fmnetnews.com

International Scleroderma Network
www.sclero.org

Irish Raynaud's and Scleroderma Society
PO Box 2958
Foxrock, Dublin 18
Ireland
(01) 235-0900
www.irishraynauds.com

Juvenile Scleroderma Network, Inc.
www.jsdn.org

Lupus Foundation of America
2000 L Street, N.W., Suite 710
Washington, D.C. 20036
(800) 558-0121
www.lupus.org

National Institute of Arthritis and Musculoskeletal and Skin Diseases (NIAMS)/ National Institutes of Health
1 AMS Circle
Bethesda, MD 20892-3675
(877) 226-4267
www.nih.gov.niams

Pulmonary Hypertension Association
850 Sligo Avenue, Suite 880
Silver Spring, MD 20910
(800) 748-7274
www.phassociation.org

Raynaud's Association, Inc.
94 Mercer Avenue
Hartsdale, NY 10530
(800) 280-8055
www.raynauds.org

Raynaud's and Scleroderma Association, UK
112 Crewe Road
Alsager, Cheshire ST7 2JA
England
01270 872776
www.raynauds.demon.co.uk

Scleroderma Clinical Trials Consortium
715 Albany Street, E-5
Boston, MA 02118
(617) 638-4486
www.sctc-online.org

Scleroderma Foundation
12 Kent Way, Suite 101
Byfield, MA 01922
(800) 722-HOPE (4673)
www.scleroderma.org

Scleroderma Research Foundation
2320 Bath Street, Suite 315
Santa Barbara, CA 93105
(800) 441-CURE (2873)
www.sclerodermaUSA.org

Scleroderma Society of Canada
95 Woodfield Road, SW
Calgary, Alberta
T2W5K5
(866) 279-0632
www.scleroderma.ca

Sjögren's Syndrome Association
8120 Woodmont Avenue
Bethesda, MD 20814
(800) 475-6473
www.sjogrens.com

Acknowledgments

FIRST AND foremost, I'd like to thank my sister, Nancy Gottesman, who helped me to gracefully enter her world and whose guidance and support allowed me to be able to actually write this book.

My profound gratitude goes to the many doctors involved in helping with this book. In particular, I'd like to thank Dr. Daniel Furst, not only for writing the foreword but for letting me tap into his extensive knowledge of scleroderma on an ongoing basis; Dr. Daniel Wallace, for continually lending both his time and technical expertise and support to the book while doing his best to keep me healthy along the way; and Dr. Philip Clements, for his dedication to the disease and willingness to help.

My love and appreciation goes to my mom, Elaine Gottesman, and my dad, George Gottesman, for their love and ongoing support since day one of my diagnosis, even while enduring their own medical odysseys.

I'd also like to thank my brother, Rick Gottesman, for his positive outlook, sound advice, and good note-taking skills.

Thanks goes out to the many scleroderma patients who so willingly shared their stories with me and allowed me to share them with you.

Special thanks and gratitude goes to Caren Berg, Jill Rosen, Vicki Anderson Granado, and Tracy Lincenberg for their ability to keep me sane as well as for their support, advice, and encouragement along the way. Also, a big thanks to those I've hounded over the years about fundraising and who have so generously donated money on my behalf.

Thanks goes to the Scleroderma Foundation and the Scleroderma Research Foundation for their ongoing commitment to helping patients and to finding a cure.

Thanks goes to Brett Grodeck, who led me to Marlowe.

And of course a heartfelt thanks goes to Maya Wirick and Evan Wirick for their infinite patience and humor, and whose delight in the book made it all worthwhile. And I can't forget K and M who were content to just let me be and write.

Lastly, thanks and gratitude goes to my publisher and editor, Matthew Lore—not only a talented editor but an incredibly nice person, too. Also, thanks goes to his associate editor, Sue McCloskey, cover designer Howard Grossman, interior page designer Pauline Neuwirth, and Peter Jacoby, as well as the rest of the Marlowe staff.

Index